Complementary and Alternative Medicine in Nursing and Midwifery

Nursing and midwifery have been at the forefront of complementary and alternative medicine (CAM) integration. Yet, the vast majority of research and commentary on CAM in nursing and midwifery fails to subject the topic to critical analysis.

Complementary and Alternative Medicine in Nursing and Midwifery brings together social science researchers from Australia, Canada, Israel, the UK and the US who are investigating the relationship and integration of CAM with nursing and midwifery. Drawing upon research experience and empirical study, contributors explore the historical, social, political and cultural facets of CAM integration with nursing and midwifery and examine the ever-expanding integration in relation to:

- the role and conceptualisation of the patient
- the role and responsibilities of different professional health care providers (nurses, midwives, alternative therapists, etc.)
- the future provision and approach of nursing and midwifery practice
- the challenges and opportunities currently facing health care systems as a result of integration.

This innovative book provides the first critical overview of this important field of health research. It is important reading for health social scientists, nurses, midwives and other health professionals as well as students in these areas with an interest in complementary and alternative medicine.

Jon Adams is Senior Lecturer at the School of Population Health, University of Queensland, Australia.
Philip Tovey is Reader in Health Sociology, School of Healthcare, University of Leeds, UK.

Researching Complementary and Alternative Medicine
J. Adams (ed.)

The Mainstreaming of Complementary and Alternative Medicine
Studies in social context
P. Tovey, G. Easthope and J. Adams (eds)

Traditional, Complementary and Alternative Medicine and Cancer Care
An international analysis of grassroots interaction
P. Tovey, J. Chatwin and A. Broom

Therapeutic Pluralism
Exploring the experiences of cancer patients and professionals
A. Broom and P. Tovey

Complementary and Alternative Medicine in Nursing and Midwifery

Towards a critical social science

Edited by Jon Adams and
Philip Tovey

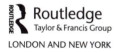

Routledge
Taylor & Francis Group

LONDON AND NEW YORK

First published 2008
by Routledge
2 Park Square, Milton Park, Abingdon, Oxon OX14 4RN

Simultaneously published in the USA and Canada
by Routledge
170 Madison Ave, New York, NY 10016

Routledge is an imprint of the Taylor & Francis Group, an informa business

Typeset in Sabon and Gill by BC Typesetting Ltd, Bristol
Printed and bound in Great Britain by
TJ International Ltd, Padstow, Cornwall

British Library Cataloguing in Publication Data
A catalogue record for this book is available from the British Library

Library of Congress Cataloging in Publication Data
Complementary and alternative medicine in nursing and midwifery:
towards a critical social science/edited by Jon Adams and Philip Tovey.
p. cm.
Includes bibliographical references and index.
ISBN-13: 978–0–415–36846–9 (hardback)
ISBN-10: 0–415–36846–4 (hardback)
ISBN-13: 978–0–415–36847–6 (pbk.)
ISBN-10: 0–415–36847–2 (pbk.)
1. Holistic nursing. 2. Midwifery. 3. Alternative medicine.
I. Adams, Jon, 1971– II. Tovey, Philip, 1963–
[DNLM: 1. Complementary Therapies–nursing.
2. Holistic Nursing–methods. 3. Midwifery–methods.
WY 86.5 C7375 2007]
RT42.C596 2007
610.73–dc22
2007008377

ISBN10: 0–415–36846–4 (hbk)
ISBN10: 0–415–36847–2 (pbk)
ISBN10: 0–203–01994–6 (ebk)

ISBN13: 978–0–415–36846–9 (hbk)
ISBN13: 978–0–415–36847–6 (pbk)
ISBN13: 978–0–203–01994–8 (ebk)

For Gorgeous Georgia – a prize chump

Contents

Contributors

Jon Adams is a Senior Lecturer in Social Science Related to Health at the School of Population Health, University of Queensland, Australia. He is also a Visiting Research Fellow at the University of Leeds, UK and is Associate Editor of the journal *Complementary Therapies in Medicine*. Jon has published extensively on different aspects of CAM and CAM research. His current research interests include the consumption and practice of CAM with reference to women's health, cancer and other chronic illness as well as the interface between CAM and general practice, nursing and midwifery.

Ivy L. Bourgeault holds the Canada Research Chair in Comparative Health Labour Policy at McMaster University, Canada. She is a member of the National Steering Committee on Rural and Remote Women's Health and of the Canadian Interdisciplinary Network for Complementary and Alternative Medicine Research. Her current research programme focuses mainly on comparative research on health occupations, but she is also involved in research on rural health care issues, with emphasis on women's health and health care, and health care providers' views of complementary and alternative medicine.

Sky E. Gross received her postgraduate degree from the Ecole des Hautes Etudes en Sciences Sociales (Paris) and is currently a PhD student at the Hebrew University of Jerusalem, Israel. Her thesis focuses on brain surgery and the relationships between biomedical and lay conceptions of the 'self'. Her publication and research background focuses on the relations between practice and knowledge, and includes fieldwork on the collaboration of complementary and biomedicine practitioners in a hospital setting; a study of the uses of alternative medicine among Israeli midwives; a historical study into psychosurgical practices; and a survey of practices of inter-disciplinary consortia in EU research programmes.

Emily Hansen is a Research Fellow in the Discipline of General Practice at the University of Tasmania, Australia. Her research interests include the social construction of medical knowledge, the relationships between professional and lay knowledge, respiratory illness and smoking, primary health care and disease prevention, gender, qualitative research and chronic illness.

Kristine A. Hirschkorn was awarded her doctorate exploring the regulation and professionalisation of herbal medicine from the Department of Sociology, McMaster University, Canada. Kristine currently holds a Canadian Institutes of Health (CIHR) Postdoctoral Fellowship at the Department of Pharmaceutical Sciences, Leslie Den Faculty of Pharmacy, University of Toronto, Canada, where she is Principal Investigator on the project 'Natural Health Products and Dietetic Practice'.

Kahryn Hughes is a Senior Research Fellow at the Institute for Health Sciences and Public Health Research, University of Leeds, UK. Her main research interests include processes of identity formation in: negotiations of definitions of care, particularly in nursing; the sociology of complementary therapies; HIV/AIDS and anorexia nervosa; and women's networks in the context of community formation.

Karen Lane is a Lecturer in the School of Social and International Studies, Deakin University, Australia. Her primary research interests are childbirth and policies related to midwifery and consumers of maternity services as well as organisational theory and discourse analysis.

Peter Morrall is Senior Lecturer in Health and Sociology at the University of Leeds, UK. His previous publications include *Murder and Society* (2006, Chichester: Wiley), *Madness and Murder* (2000, London: Whurr) and *Sociology and Nursing* (2001, London: Routledge). He is currently writing a book on the sociology of counselling/psychotherapy. Peter's theoretical heritage embraces scepticism, realism, and polemics. He is also a restless traveller, rabid vegetarian, and fiddles with the saxophone.

Judith T. Shuval is Professor Emerita in the Department of Sociology and Anthropology, Hebrew University of Jerusalem, Israel. Her research interests focus upon the sociology of health and health care in Israel, alternative health care in Israel, the planning of health manpower, and the occupational integration of Russian immigrant physicians to Israel.

Philip Tovey is Reader in Health Sociology, School of Healthcare, University of Leeds, UK. His main research interests relate to the sociological aspects of CAM in cancer care, the appropriation of CAM by nursing, and the intersection of indigenous traditional medicines with globalised CAM in poorer countries.

Paaige K. Turner is Associate Professor and Director of Graduate Studies, Department of Communication, Saint Louis University, Missouri, USA. She conducts research in the general areas of organisational communication, feminist theory and health communication. Her research to date has examined the creation and negotiation of contradiction, specifically within the topics of organisational socialisation, midwifery and birth and the body in the workplace.

Acknowledgements

Chapter 2 in this collection has been previously published in a modified form as Turner, P. (2004) Mainstreaming alternative medicine: doing midwifery at the intersection. *Qualitative Health Research* 14(5): 644–62. We are grateful to Sage Publications for the permission to republish this paper in modified form.

Chapter 4 in this collection has been previously published in modified form as Tovey, P. and Adams, J. (2003) Nostalgic and nostophobic referencing and the authentication of nurses' use of complementary therapies. *Social Science & Medicine* 56(7): 1469–80. We are grateful to Elsevier for the permission to republish this paper in modified form.

Abbreviations

AARN	Alberta Association of Registered Nurses
ACHN	Australian College of Holistic Nurses
AMA	Australian Medical Association
ANMC	Australian Nursing and Midwifery Council
APN	advanced practice nurse
BMA	British Medical Association
CAM	complementary and alternative medicine
CNM	certified nurse-midwife
CT	computerised tomographic
FDA	Food and Drug Administration
GMC	General Medical Council
GP	general practitioner
IV	intravenous
MHRA	Medicines and Healthcare products Regulatory Agency
MRSA	methicillin-resistant staphylococcus aureus
NCCAM	National Centre for Complementary and Alternative Medicine
NEHSL	National Electronic Health Service Library
NHS	National Health Service
NMB	Nurses and Midwives Board New South Wales
NMC	Nursing and Midwifery Council
NZCOM	New Zealand College of Midwives
PCO	primary care organisation
RCN	Royal College of Nursing
RCNA	Royal College of Nursing Australia
RCT	randomised controlled trial
SAS	Sense About Science
SCST	Select Committee on Science and Technology
SWT	social worlds theory
UKCC	United Kingdom Central Council for Nursing, Midwifery and Health

Introduction: Towards a critical social science of CAM in nursing and midwifery

Jon Adams and Philip Tovey

Within the last decade there have been significant developments in the relationship between complementary and alternative medicine (CAM)[1] and biomedical provision. Rhetorics of integration have become increasingly commonplace and an air of consensus, about the incorporation of CAM, as an accompaniment or supplement to conventional treatments, has become apparent. Regardless of the potential barriers to successful integration (Barrett 2003; Hughes 2004; Coulter 2004) the rising tide of popularity of these medicines amongst both providers and consumers has helped cement CAM as a key public health and health care/provision issue (Bodeker and Kronenberg 2002; Giordano et al. 2003). But with the emergence of consensus comes the potential for a less critical and distanced analysis of the integrative process. This is a tendency, we argue, that should be resisted.

As the mainstreaming of CAM has gathered momentum (Tovey et al. 2004), so too has the interest and activity of the research community. Accompanying clinical investigation – aiming to assess the efficacy of CAM treatments (Katchup 2002; Pirotta 2007) – has blossomed a wide range of disciplinary approaches and methodological designs which aim to explore and explain different dimensions of CAM and integration (Adams 2007).

Such research effort has involved biostatisticians (Sibbritt 2007), public health researchers (Bodeker and Kronenberg 2002; Dew and Carroll 2007), medical geographers (Andrews et al. 2004), CAM practitioner-researchers (Hope-Allen et al. 2004; Steinsbekk 2007) plus many others. A significant part of this has been a broadly conceived sociology of CAM (Tovey and Adams 2002; Tovey et al. 2004). A particular strength of much (though not all) of this work has been the capacity to stand aside from advocacy or attack and consider CAM in its own right – as a social process.

The bulk of this sociological study to date has tended to concentrate upon the relations between CAM and the medical profession (Adams 2001; 2006; Siahpush 2000). Although this focus has helped unearth a number of significant findings it has also hidden other important issues and developments from the sociological gaze (Adams 2004). One area of development that has until recently escaped such attention has been the growing affinity with, support for, and practice of CAM within nursing and midwifery.

A range of surveys, albeit often illustrating varying designs and degrees of methodological rigour (Leach 2002), have identified high levels of support for and practice of CAM amongst nurses and midwives in numerous countries and settings (Allaire et al. 2000; Brolinson et al. 2001; Leach 2002; Rankin-Box 1997; Hunt et al. 2004; Rooney et al. 2001; Sohn and Loveland Cook 2002; Wilkinson and Simpson 2002; Tracy et al. 2003; McPartland and Pruit 1999). Alongside such practitioner interest and involvement have appeared a number of policy and practice guidelines and statements from formal nursing and midwifery representative bodies in a number of countries (AARN 2000; RCNA 1997; NMB 2006; NZCOM 2000). Even when variations in the territory, identity and standing of the professions are acknowledged (both across health care systems and in many cases between nursing and midwifery within the same system of health care) these professions do appear to be at the forefront of CAM integration.

The vast majority, if not all, of the early research on CAM and nursing and midwifery has been authored by spokespeople, researchers and practitioners from within the two professions themselves (for a more detailed analysis of such insider claims and perspectives see Tovey and Adams Chapter 4 this collection). This monopoly, while providing a useful impetus to internal debate on CAM within nursing and midwifery, is by its very nature limited in scope (coming from advocates) and tends to omit elements crucial to a distanced, critical research agenda on CAM.

First, the insider perspective advances and thereby fails to problematise the taken-for-granted assumptions of the culture of nursing and midwifery more generally; nursing advocates of CAM integration have tended not to present a critical perspective to inquiry or reflection, instead *assuming* the appropriateness and benefits of continued alignment with CAM (Adams and Tovey 2004).

Second, and related to this lack of critical perspective, has been a failure of previous authors (from within the ranks of nursing and midwifery) to acknowledge and explore the true importance of the nature and location of the two professions. Their historical development as well as their current structural and cultural positions are all core features underpinning an understanding of the changing relationship between nursing and midwifery and a range of CAM.

If we subject the relationship between CAM and nursing and midwifery to closer historical, cultural and political analysis, two fundamental features of the health care landscape become evident. To begin with, it is important that investigators at least acknowledge the range of sub-groupings within these two professions. These are constructed along the lines of types of provision (e.g. privately or publicly funded), political or philosophical schools of practice (e.g. postmodern nursing) or sub-specialisms based upon care settings (e.g. critical care nursing, palliative care nursing, aged care nursing, etc.).

In addition, variations between some CAM modalities and approaches must also be borne in mind when examining the relationships between these medicines and conventional health care practitioners. While a number of groupings have been proposed with which to classify the range of CAM (e.g. NCCAM 2002) the underlying commonality across therapies and treatments is often no more than the exclusion from conventional medical practice and education.

Book structure and content

There is a long record of researching nursing and midwifery within health social science (Willis 1983; Davis-Floyd and Sargent 1996). And as we have already noted a not insignificant body of work has been established on CAM. Only very recently, though, has an approach and framework been offered with which to plan and guide ongoing and future co-ordinated social science investigation of CAM in direct relation to nursing and/or midwifery (Adams and Tovey 2004; Tovey and Adams 2002). This framework, introducing a number of core research domains for critical investigation, has provided the impetus and structure for the present collection.

Following that broad structure which we have detailed elsewhere (Tovey and Adams 2002), this book is divided into three parts: inter-professional issues; intra-professional issues; and, public health and patient issues. Of course, in practice these areas are not mutually exclusive; overlap in the issues arising is inevitable. The split does, however, provide us with a useful framing device.

Part I, inter-professional issues, is important for two reasons: it acknowledges, first, that nursing and midwifery operate within a network of disciplinary relationships. And, second, that changes to the character of CAM – in this case the incorporation of non-biomedical therapeutic options – may well impinge (positively or negatively) on those relationships. In the opening chapter, Bourgeault and Hirschkorn explain how there is a paucity of research that compares knowledge, attitudes and behaviours towards CAM across different mainstream provider groups and in response the authors outline a qualitative study of physicians, nurses and midwives in two Canadian provinces. The data from this study reveals discrepancies between professionals' views and actions, identifies a hierarchy of openness and illustrates shifting attitudes and behaviours over time across the three mainstream provider groups with regard to CAM.

In Chapter 2, Turner provides a case study of the intersection of conventional and alternative birth care practices in the USA. The chapter considers the experiences of one group of alternative birth care providers (using CAM) within the wider socio-political sphere, examining the relationship of these alternative providers with conventional medicine.

The first part closes with a polemic by Morrall (Chapter 3). Writing as a sociologist with a nursing background he considers the question of the relationship between CAM and the occupational status of both medicine and nursing. Morrall looks at what he describes as the credibility of CAM (in relation to evidence) and the validity of critiquing CAM from outside of its epistemological framework. He then looks at the different positions of nursing and medicine *vis-à-vis* the potential impact of CAM on their occupational status. Provocatively, it is argued that the occupational status of nursing is most likely to be hindered by the association with CAM and that a better strategy would be to focus on the unglamorous but essential aspects of basic patient care.

In Part II we turn to the intra-professional issues (within nursing and midwifery) introduced by an association with CAM. The part opens with a chapter (4) by Tovey and Adams which reports on research examining the way in which writers – within the CAM nursing sub-world – adopt a recourse to history as a strategy to authenticate the relationship between nursing and CAM and so facilitate continuing integration. The authors argue that these rhetorical strategies can be understood in the context of the need to engage in (primarily though not exclusively) intra-professional persuasion: to protect and develop the values of their nursing sub-world (with its distinctive connotations for the development of nursing) over alternatives within the profession.

In Chapter 5, Hughes, continuing the theme of intra-professional dynamics, looks at the integration of CAM therapies in relation to broader notions of care and holism with which CAM is so closely related. The chapter is based on empirical evidence from two studies conducted in the UK. The author examines how the meanings of care and holism are used to hold off and differentiate both individual identity and professional boundaries (the latter a theme returned to in the following chapter). Hughes argues that debates about CAM nursing care relate closely to broader work on the sociology of care; she considers the opportunity for a critical engagement between the two developing bodies of knowledge.

The third and final chapter (6) of this part is a comparative study of nurses and midwives practising CAM in Israel. The authors, Shuval and Gross, build on their earlier work which has considered the negotiative processes of boundary crossing to consider nurses and midwives using CAM. Again, this data is considered within the framework offered by Boundary Studies. Approaching the analysis with an emphasis on within-profession variation, the chapter considers not only differences between the two groups but also differences within both nursing and midwifery respectively.

The final part of the collection moves away from considering CAM integration in predominantly professional terms to explore aspects of CAM in nursing and midwifery with a view to their impact upon the role and care of consumers/patients and/or broader notions of public health. In Chapter 7, Lane, focusing attention upon 'latent' and 'realised' risk cultures, argues that 'woman-centred care' within midwifery practice is inherently compatible with CAM and its integration within the midwifery field. As Lane explains, the fusion of these two practice developments provides midwives with the opportunity to promote themselves as primary care givers as well as signifying the individualisation of health care and the recent shift towards consumerism whereby women/mothers are facilitated to take greater participation in their health care decision-making.

The closing chapter of this part and the book (Chapter 8, Hansen) critically analyses the relationship between holistic wellness nursing (closely linked to CAM practices and approaches to health) and the new public health. Hansen explores the relevance of the socio-cultural critique closely aligned to the new public health for holistic wellness nursing. She suggests that a greater awareness about this critique may serve to stimulate debate among holistic wellness nurses regarding the potential challenges of victim-blaming and oppressive representations of a healthy or well self associated with the wellness movement.

The chapters in this collection provide an overview of investigation currently being undertaken on CAM in nursing and midwifery from within the social sciences. The wider body of social science literature/scholarship focusing upon this specific aspect of CAM integration remains relatively small scale (especially when considered alongside more conventional substantive areas of nursing and midwifery receiving research attention) and readers will be hard-pressed to locate similar published research beyond that outlined in this book.

There is much benefit to be gleaned from subjecting CAM in nursing and midwifery to critical social science examination and as this collection illustrates social scientists in various parts of the world have initiated the early empirical and conceptual groundwork necessary to develop an exciting and fruitful research programme on the topic. Our hope as editors (and authors) is that this collection provokes debate and stimulates further research interest upon CAM in nursing and midwifery – there are certainly a vast range of pertinent research questions still to be addressed, all of which can only be strengthened by the inclusion of critical approaches and analyses as provided by the disciplines of the social sciences.

Note

1 Here we refer to those practices, technologies and medications not traditionally part of conventional care and including acupuncture, aromatherapy, chiropractic, homeopathy, hypnotherapy, spiritual healing, reflexology, massage therapy, osteopathy, reiki healing, music and art therapy among others. It is acknowledged that

the definition of complementary and alternative medicine is both temporally and spatially variable and the subject of considerable contestation. Nevertheless, in line with the vast majority of academic writers in the field the term and its acronym CAM are used throughout this book.

References

AARN (Alberta Association of Registered Nurses) (2000) *Alternative and/or Complementary Therapy: Standards for Registered Nurses*. Edmonton: AARN.

Adams, J. (2001) Direct integrative practice, time constraints and reactive strategy: an examination of general practitioner therapists' perceptions of their complementary medicine. *Journal of Management in Medicine* 15(4): 312–22.

Adams, J. (2004) Examining the sites of interface between CAM and conventional health care: extending the sociological gaze. *Complementary Therapies in Medicine* 12: 69–70.

Adams, J. (2006) The use of complementary and alternative medicines within hospital midwifery: models of care and professional struggle. *Complementary Therapies in Clinical Practice* 12(1): 40–7.

Adams J. (ed.) (2007) *Researching Complementary and Alternative Medicine*. London: Routledge.

Adams, J. and Tovey, P. (2004) CAM and nursing: from advocacy to critical sociology. In Tovey, P., Easthope, G. and Adams, J. (eds) *The Mainstreaming of Complementary and Alternative Medicine: Studies in Social Context*. London: Routledge, pp. 158–74.

Allaire, A. D., Moos, M.-K. and Wells, S. R. (2000) Complementary and alternative medicine in pregnancy: a survey of North Carolina certified nurse-midwives. *Obstetrics and Gynecology* 95: 19–23.

Andrews, G.J., Wiles, J. and Miller, K. (2004) The geography of complementary medicine: perspectives and prospects. *Complementary Therapies in Nursing and Midwifery* 10: 175–85.

Barrett, B. (2003) Alternative, complementary, and conventional medicine: is integration upon us? *Journal of Alternative and Complementary Medicine* 9(3): 417–27.

Bodeker, G. and Kronenberg, A. (2002) A public health agenda for traditional, complementary and alternative medicine. *American Journal of Public Health* 92(10): 1582–90.

Brolinson, P. G., Price, J. H., Ditmyer, M. and Reis, D. (2001) Nurses' perceptions of complementary and alternative medical therapies. *Journal of Community Health* 26(3): 175–89.

Coulter, I. (2004) Integration and paradigm clash: the practical difficulties of integrative medicine. In Tovey, P., Easthope, G. and Adams, J. (eds) *The Mainstreaming of Complementary and Alternative Medicine: Studies in Social Context*. London: Routledge, pp. 103–22.

Davis-Floyd, R. and Sargent, C. (1996) The social production of authoritative knowledge in pregnancy and childbirth. *Medical Anthropology* 10(2): 111–20.

Dew, K. and Carroll, P. (2007) Public health and CAM: exploring overlap, contrast and dissonance. In Adams, J. (ed.) *Researching Complementary and Alternative Medicine*. London: Routledge, pp. 117–32.

Giordano, J., Garcia, M. K. and Klein, K. (2003) Complementary and alternative medicine in mainstream public health: a role for research in fostering integration. *Journal of Alternative and Complementary Medicine* 9(3): 441–5.

Hope-Allan, N., Adams, J., Sibbritt, D. and Tracy, S. (2004) The use of acupuncture in maternity care: a pilot study evaluating the acupuncture service in an Australian hospital antenatal clinic. *Complementary Therapies in Nursing and Midwifery* 10(4): 229–32.

Hughes, K. (2004) Health as individual responsibility: possibilities and personal struggle. In Tovey, P., Easthope, G. and Adams, J. (eds) *The Mainstreaming of Complementary and Alternative Medicine: Studies in Social Context*. London: Routledge, pp. 25–46.

Hunt, V., Randle, J. and Freshwater, D. (2004) Paediatric nurses' attitudes to massage and aromatherapy massage. *Complementary Therapies in Nursing and Midwifery* 10(3): 194–201.

Katchup, T. J. (2002) Acupuncture: theory, efficacy and practice. *Annals of Internal Medicine* 136(5): 374–83.

Leach M. J. (2002) Public, nurse and medical practitioner attitude and practice of natural medicine. *Complementary Therapies in Nursing and Midwifery* 10: 13–21.

McPartland, J. M. and Pruit, P. L. (1999) Opinions of MDs, RNs, allied health practitioners towards osteopathic medicine and alternative therapies: results from a Vermont survey. *Journal of the American Osteopathic Association* 99(2): 101–8.

NCCAM (National Centre for Complementary and Alternative Medicine) (2002) *What is Complementary and Alternative Medicine?* Bethesda, Md: NCCAM.

NMB (Nurses and Midwives Board New South Wales) (2006) *Complementary Therapies in Nursing and Midwifery Practice*: www.nmb.nsw.gov.au/complementary-therapies/default.aspx

NZCOM (New Zealand College of Midwives) (2000) *Consensus Statement, Complementary Therapies*. Wellington: NZCOM.

Pirotta, M. (2007) Towards the application of RCTs for CAM: methodological challenges. In Adams, J. (ed.) *Researching Complementary and Alternative Medicine*. London: Routledge, pp. 52–71.

Rankin-Box, D. (1997) Therapies in practice: a survey assessing nurses' use of complementary therapies. *Complementary Therapies in Nursing and Midwifery* 3(4): 92–9.

RCNA (Royal College of Nursing Australia) (1997) *Position Statement, Complementary Therapies in Nursing*. Canberra: RCNA.

Rooney, B., Fiocco, G., Hughes, P. and Halter, S. (2001) Provider attitudes and use of alternative medicine in a Midwestern medical practice in 2001. *Wisconson Medical Journal* 100(7): 27–31.

Schroeder, C. A. and Likkel, J. (1999) Integrative health care: the revolution is upon us. *Public Health Nursing* 16(4): 233–4.

Siahpush, M. (2000) A critical review of the sociology of alternative medicine: research on users, practitioners and the orthodoxy. *Health* 4(2): 159–78.

Sibbritt, D. (2007) Utilising existing data sets for CAM consumption research: the case of cohort studies. In Adams, J. (ed.) *Researching Complementary and Alternative Medicine*. London: Routledge, pp. 37–51.

Sohn, P. M. and Loveland Cook, C. A. (2002) Nurse practitioner knowledge of complementary and alternative health care: foundation for practice. *Journal of Advanced Nursing* 39(1): 9–16.

Steinsbekk, A. (2007) The practitioner as researcher: research capacity building within the ranks of CAM. In Adams, J. (ed.) *Researching Complementary and Alternative Medicine*. London: Routledge, pp. 105–16.

Tovey, P. and Adams, J. (2002) Towards a sociology of CAM and nursing. *Complementary Therapies in Nursing and Midwifery* 8(1): 12–16.

Tovey, P., Easthope, G. and Adams, J. (eds) (2004) *The Mainstreaming of Complementary and Alternative Medicine: Studies in Social Context*. London: Routledge.

Tracy, M. F., Lindquist, R., Watanuki, S., Sendelbach, S., Kreitzer, M. J, Berman, B. and Savik, K. (2003) Nurse attitudes towards the use of complementary and alternative therapies in critical care. *Heart and Lung* 32(3): 197–209.

Wilkinson, J. M. and Simpson, M. D. (2002) Personal and professional use of complementary therapies by nurses in NSW, Australia. *Complementary Therapies in Nursing and Midwifery* 8(3): 142–7.

Willis, E. (1983) *Medical Dominance: The Division of Labour in Australian Health Care*. Sydney: George Allen and Unwin.

Part I

Inter-professional issues

Chapter 1

CAM integration in inter-professional context

Nursing, midwifery and medicine in Canada

Ivy L. Bourgeault and Kristine A. Hirschkorn

Introduction

A spate of previous articles over the last decade has addressed mainstream health care professionals' knowledge, attitudes and behaviour regarding complementary and alternative medicine (CAM). Nevertheless, there is a paucity of research: comparing this issue across provider groups and settings (Baugniet et al, 2000; Burg et al. 1998; Straub and Henley 2000; Tovey 1997); that has utilised qualitative methods for greater depth of analysis (Adams 2000; Bernstein and Shuval 1997; Bourgeault 1996; Fitch et al. 1999; Gray et al. 1998; Goldner 2000; Montbriand 2000; Sakala 1988; Verhoef et al. 2002); and even less that draws upon any sort of conceptual framework or theoretical perspective (Adams 2000; Adams and Tovey 2001; Bourgeault 1996; Tovey and Adams 2001; 2002; 2003). This has severely limited our ability to collectively advance understanding in this field of study. In this chapter, we attempt to address some of the limitations of this literature through a comparative examination of the knowledge, attitudes and behaviour of physicians, nurses and midwives regarding CAM in two Canadian provinces – British Columbia and Ontario. We also draw upon existing theoretical contributions to the area of CAM more generally (Saks 1996; 2000; Sharma 2000; Siahpush 1999; Tovey and Adams 2002).

Comparing mainstream professionals' perspectives on CAM

Much of the research that is available on health care professionals' views of CAM focuses on physicians' perspectives, due presumably to the apparent discrepancy in their views and those of CAM providers, but also because physicians hold a great deal of power in defining the terms and conditions under which CAM may be practised. A survey of English language literature reveals that physicians in 'developed' nations demonstrate both tolerance for and a moderate interest in CAM but no apparent increase in the perception of its usefulness (cf. Adams 2000; Astin et al. 1998; Berman et al. 1998;

1999; 2002; Bernstein and Shuval 1997; Borkan et al. 1994; Botting and Cook 2000; Chen et al. 1999; Cohen and Eisenberg 2002; Eisenberg et al. 1998; Goldner 2000; Gray et al. 1998; Hasan et al. 2000; Tovey 1997). Summarising across these studies, we can conclude, at minimum, that most physicians express a need for more information and reliable studies. Furthermore, many adopt an attitude of acceptance of patients' choices and at least half believe in the value of at least one CAM modality. An equivalent number refer patients to alternative practitioners, although very few actually practise any form of CAM (Adams 2004). Canadian physicians have not been found to be atypical in this regard (Bourgeault 1996; Curry and Smith 1998; Goldszmidt et al. 1995; Verhoef et al. 2002; Verhoef and Sutherland 1995a; 1995b).

A growing number of articles focus on the views of nurses regarding CAM, identifying both an interest in evaluating CAM and support for a minimal nursing role as educator/information provider/counsellor for patients (Adams and Tovey 2001; DeKeyser et al. 2001; Frisch 2001a; 2001b; Johnson 2000; King et al. 1999; Lorenzo 2003; Mayer et al. 2001; Montbriand 2000; Salmenpera et al. 1998; Taylor 2002; Tovey and Adams 2003; Trevelyan 1996; Wilkinson and Simpson 2002). Indeed, in line with the holistic focus towards nursing care, the profession has been perceived as 'naturally' more responsive towards the use of various CAM modalities. Many nurses use CAM in their work, with aromatherapy and massage being the most popular, followed by therapeutic touch. The one published study of nurses in Canada (Fitch et al. 1999) similarly found they express an open attitude towards and indicate the need for information regarding CAM. These nurses also appear to have an interest in communicating with patients about their use – more so than identified among physicians. Unfortunately, very few of these articles involve primary research whereby nurses have been interviewed or surveyed regarding their opinions and behaviour. These papers do, however, draw attention to the link between holistic nursing, patient-centred care models and CAM, many suggesting that nursing is well situated to undertake a central role in patient education, and to a lesser extent, in delivery of CAM.

Much less is known of other health care professionals, such as midwives, regarding CAM (Adams 2006; Allaire et al. 2000; Dimond 1998; Raisler 2000; Sakala 1988; Silverman 1995; Taylor 2002; Tiran and Mack 2000). Perhaps this is due to how in some jurisdictions, such as Canada and to some extent in the United States, midwives continue to be considered akin to alternative practitioners themselves despite being well integrated into maternity care systems worldwide. Alternately, midwives may not be considered sufficiently distinct from nursing to warrant specific analysis. Whatever the case, what we do know is that there is an increasing interest among midwives towards CAM, with the most widely used modality being aromatherapy (Adams 2006; Burns et al. 2000a; 2000b; Burns and Blamey 1994;

Rose 1994; Smith 1991; Tiran and Mack 2000). A UK survey conducted in 1997 indicated that midwives were the highest users of CAM among all professional groups (34%) (Tiran and Mack 2000). Even higher rates of usage – over 90% – have been reported of independent (i.e. non-nurse) midwives in the US (Allaire et al. 2000; Sakala 1988), but the limited geographical range and particular political contexts of these two studies may impose limitations on generalising or transferring these findings to broader populations. To date, no study of CAM among Canadian midwives has been reported in the published literature.

Overall, the picture that emerges from this literature is that nurses and midwives appear much more open towards CAM than physicians, but admittedly there is very little empirical evidence to demonstrate this systematically. Glaus (1988) was one of the first authors to comment on how 'nursing care is the constant intermediate between school and alternative medicine' (p. 250) and further that there was a growing trend (at least in the European context they examined) 'toward a greater separation between school medicine and nursing than between alternative medicine and nursing' (p. 250). Part of this trend was attributed by Glaus to increasing patient interest and in turn the closer relations nurses tend to have with patients.

Tovey (1997) examined the difference between provider groups more systematically in a large-scale study of non-orthodox practitioners in the UK. He argues that although there has been an overall liberalisation of attitudes among mainstream professionals *vis-à-vis* CAM, this is not necessarily generalisable across provider groups. Specifically, he found that 'there is a schism within orthodoxy on this issue and that schism is occupationally based: at the extremes, consultants [i.e. medical specialists] remain characteristically dismissive of alternative practitioners, nurses overwhelmingly enthusiastic' (p. 1129). Further, Tovey found that the nature of the CAM modality being considered was of little significance but rather the differentiation was within orthodoxy. Another comparative study focusing upon health science faculty members in Florida found that while 52% of medicine faculty reported using CAM (mirroring usage in the general population), usage was much higher among nursing faculty (74%) (Burg et al. 1998). Straub and Henley (2000) surveyed physicians in several specialisations and advanced practice nurses (APNs) regarding their views of CAM practice, CAM effectiveness, patients' use and CAM education. They found that physicians were the least likely to offer CAM therapies, whereas nurses were most likely to offer chiropractic, herbal medicine, or acupuncture.

Similar findings are reported in Canada. Specifically, Montbriand (2000) reports that Canadian 'nurses were about twice as likely as other professionals [physicians and pharmacists] to be users of alternative therapies, but were half as likely to suggest these products or therapies to patients' (p. 23). This is an interesting discrepancy which may point to the influences of broader structural barriers to professional referral to CAM. She does, however, note that there was a general association between practitioners who did not suggest CAM to patients and negative attitudes towards CAM. Another Canadian study focused on the views of a variety of students in health professional programmes including medicine, nursing, physiotherapy, occupational therapy and pharmacy (Baugniet et al. 2000). It was found that compared to medical students, nurses are more likely to have consulted a CAM practitioner, report more knowledge about CAM as well as hold more positive attitudes towards CAM.

Thus, similar to what we find in the non-comparative literature, the major trend in these comparative studies is that the philosophy and practice of nursing (and we will argue here midwifery as well – cf. Adams 2006) is amenable to CAM and thus less problematic. There is an implicit assumption in much of this literature that because they are less powerful groups nurses and midwives are therefore less 'oppositionary'. This assumption would appear to translate into their also being less of a focus of study. Physicians' practices and paradigms of practice are viewed as inherently more contradictory (and the power relation between them and CAM practitioners most discrepant). What is less clear from the literature are the reasons why this might be the case. We turn now to the more conceptually based literature to provide some insights in this regard.

Inter-professional relations

As part of their development of a sociology of CAM and nursing, Tovey and Adams (2002) highlight how 'given that nursing practice is located within a web of professional interaction there is much to be gained from work that seeks to explicitly explore various points of interface with other stakeholders' (p. 13). This argument can be extended to other health professions including medicine and midwifery. Tovey and Adams (2002) further identify a number of intersections with nursing practice such as: the relations between nursing and medicine; the complex relations between nursing and lay CAM practitioners; the intersection between nursing and health management; and the relationship between nursing and location (i.e. the relevance of the health care system and location in the private or voluntary sector).

These intersections as identified by Tovey and Adams parallel some of the key concepts from the broader sociological literature on the professions. For example, Freidson (1970) outlines how medical dominance consists of a variety of levels of influence including the control over the content and context of medical work, control over other health professions and over patients. Likewise, others have acknowledged that professions do not exist in a vacuum, but rather in relationship to one another, both in the workplace as well as on a broader structural level (Abbott 1988).

Given the far-reaching effects of status relations and jurisdictional boundaries among professions, it is surprising that these insights have thus far
largely escaped analyses of professionals' behaviours regarding CAM, with
only a few exceptions. Tovey (1997: 1132), for example, points out that
'the unequal distribution of autonomy, authority and financial reward
within orthodoxy' supports the notion of what he refers to as a *status
related schism*: a greater flexibility to the non-orthodox being expressed
among those least effectively rewarded by the existing arrangements'.
Tovey argues further that the affinity between nurses and alternative medicine might also be related to a gendered compatibility. Adams and Tovey
(2001: 138) further highlight the use of strategies that 'naturalise CAM to
the nursing environment' and how 'CAM practice provides nurses with an
opportunity to distance themselves from a range of specific (and negatively
interpreted) features of conventional medicine'. In addition to this 'distancing' strategy, they argue that CAM is utilised to advance nursing: 'as a
dynamic and flexible profession with CAM integration portrayed as an
opportunity for nurses to be proactive and to drive change in healthcare'
(Adams and Tovey 2001: 138).

Inter-professional status differentials have also been found to influence
midwives' behaviour. Tiran (2003), for example, points out that, erroneously,
'many midwives are under the impression that they are not allowed to
administer or advise on [CAM] if the obstetric medical staff disagree, but
this is simply not the case' (Tiran 2003: 12). Sakala (1988) also notes the
hostility that Utah midwives have faced from medical personnel due to
their being perceived as fringe practitioners.

In our study (outlined below in more detail), such inter-professional
tensions between nurses and physicians and between midwives and physicians emerged as a strong theme. Many nurses and midwives found themselves tempering their CAM-related behaviour to suit physicians or even
engaging in strategies to 'convert' physicians or openly normalise CAM-
related treatment.

Methodology

This chapter draws upon findings from interviews with a total of 41 participants (13 physicians, 16 nurses and 12 midwives) conducted between June
and December 2003. Ontario and British Columbia were chosen as the
research sites as all three provider groups practise in a regulated environment in both provinces. Although both provinces are home to a variety of
CAM providers and modalities, British Columbia is generally regarded as
being a more hospitable environment for CAM (as least *vis-à-vis* the
public) than it is in Ontario. Semi-structured interviews were conducted
with each of the professionals in the two research settings. This allowed

the professionals to explain their views at length and to highlight the most salient issues of concern to them.

Efforts were made to include a range of professionals working in a variety of structural contexts (e.g. staff, managers, educators in institutions and community-based practices). Specifically, in the physician group, this range included specialists (e.g. oncology etc.) and family/general practitioners. In the nursing group, this range included those working as nurse practitioners and teaching in these programmes as well as hospital and public health-based professionals and educators. Midwives included those attending home and hospital births, those working pre- and post-regulation, as well as some (previously) trained as nurses.[1]

Comparing influences on the attitudes and behaviours of physicians, nurses and midwives

What they think about CAM

There was variability expressed both within and between professional groups regarding attitudes towards CAM use and integration. Two very different opinions of physicians are nicely exemplified in the following two quotes:

> It would be nice if patients could feel like all the different providers were working together . . . It would be nice if we were all a bit more informed about it too. Integration I guess breeds understanding. It would be nice if we were a bit more up to date on what kinds of therapy are available and what the evidence is for them and how they're used.
>
> (Physician)

> I would do everything that I could to stand in the way of [integrating CAM into our system], unless they were proven.
>
> (Physician)

Some of this variability could be attributed to personal preferences but other influences on attitudes identified by our medical respondents included medical specialty and the related context within which physicians practised. For example, one physician stated:

> Within oncology I think people are probably a bit more open minded maybe than the average physician just because in oncology, you get faced frequently with patients where . . . you don't have a treatment to offer them that's going to help, so you really have to, I think, be open minded to their own needs for looking beyond conventional medicine.

So I would think in oncology they would be a bit more accepting for complementary therapies.

(Physician)

There was less variability expressed by the nursing respondents with most displaying positive attitudes towards CAM. The following quote is exemplary in this regard:

I think there are more and more mainstream practitioners like me who realise that this has a lot of benefits, and . . . like the College of Nurses, actually has guidelines for nurses practising using complementary therapies. . . . I've never separated the two in my mind. I mean holistic nursing includes things like CAM. Because how can you be holistic if you leave out a whole big area of health care?

(Nurse)

Although little variability in attitude was identified among our own respondents, some of the nurses did acknowledge that differences do exist in nurses' opinions:

I'm more open to different therapies . . . but I know I've had nurses challenge me and say 'How do you live with yourself if you think you can sit there and recommend to nursing students that complementary therapies are good?' And I say 'well I'm not saying they're good. I'm saying we need to acknowledge our patients are using them and we need to have discussions with our patients about that and it's not our role to say yes that's good, [no] that's bad'.

(Nurse)

The midwives interviewed also spoke of the variability that existed within their profession with respect to various CAM modalities:

Some people will be very passionate about it and feel that it's absolutely germane to midwifery practices and others who may sit more in the kind of views that I have which is that it's an easy accompaniment but it's not germane to practice.

(Midwife)

Acknowledging that there may be variability within midwifery, comments from all of our respondents led us to believe that midwives' views were on a different scale than those of physicians and nurses. That is, the range of views within midwifery tended to be more positive than nursing, which in turn tended to be more positive than medicine. It must be noted, however, that without a random sample of all practitioners, this is difficult to say for certain.

Our informants were not only forthright in their opinions of fellow colleagues, they also had strong views of the way in which other health professionals approach CAM use and integration. This also lends support to our supposed hierarchy of views from less positive to most positive from physicians to nurses to midwives. For example, one physician commented that

> I think the nurses are more informed. I think they . . . know more what the patients are taking and what the current trend or the current products that are being used are. And they're more hooked into the non-pharmacologic or non-medication complementary therapies. They know where patients can go for those things and I think a lot of prac- titioners of, for example, therapeutic touch are nurses etc. So they're more hooked in.
>
> (Physician)

So not only are nurses considered by physicians to be more positive, these views are linked to nurses' close relationship with patients. Both our nurse and medical respondents also thought this to be the case for midwives; speci- fically that their close relationship with clients reflected more accepting atti- tudes towards CAM practices.

As we asked for clarification of their views of other health care profes- sionals, several of the comments by physicians highlight the role scientific training plays:

> I don't think [nurses] are particularly more vulnerable than doctors. They don't have the same level of training to be critical but sometimes I'm not so sure about the level of training we're providing our docs from that point of view, [in terms of] critically assessing evidence.
>
> (Physician)

> I would prefer to believe that there's some sort of correlation between a background science and scepticism about this thing.
>
> (Physician)

Some nurses were also affected by the level of evidence supporting CAM:

> If we eventually get to the stage where we have evidence that supports that CAM is effective either on its own or in combination with more standard practice produces better patient outcomes, then I think that would be great to have that integrated into practice.
>
> (Nurse)

Perhaps more consistent with physicians' views of nurses, one expressed a more reflexive view of evidence:

> the evidence that they would look at would include realising the limits of evidence regarding mainstream therapies. . . . I mean there's nobody [that] ever did a randomised controlled trial of putting women up in stirrups . . . So you know kind of the clay feet of conventional medicine and that maybe . . . makes you more open to complementary and alternative side because it's like well not quite accepting that double standard as much as you know.
>
> (Nurse)

This more reflexive view is what made another more willing to support patients' choices:

> I think that the best thing we can do . . . is have our patients make as informed a choice as possible. So directing them to resources that . . . we consider credible, and again that's credible from a . . . conventional perspective. And I actually think that it's important for many patients to maintain their hope, to maintain a sense of control over their health care to use these therapies. I think there's value in them. It may not be value that we would acknowledge with a lot of our randomised clinical trials but there's a lot of I think psychosocial benefits for patients using complementary therapies.
>
> (Nurse)

Some nurses also expressed concerns about the integration of CAM and its impact on the 'scientific' rigour of the CAM modality:

> I have some concerns that some of the things that are happening in terms of you know, [they] have randomised clinical trials, test out these therapies, and see if they 'work'. And that's work in quotations. Because they're using a standard that's very much a biomedical standard. And then if it 'works', we will then co-opt that therapy and prescribe it within our clinical settings. And I think that a lot of therapies could be disempowered by having them removed from the paradigms and philosophies in which they were developed.
>
> (Nurse)

Both nurses and physicians suggested that midwives' views were even less conservative. For example, one nurse stated emphatically that:

> Midwives are feistier as a whole. They're more likely to challenge the system. They're less accepting of medical approaches. . . . I think that

nurses as a whole are a little more comfortable with mainstream medical than complementary and alternative although there [are] obviously exceptions.

(Nurse)

Midwives in turn had their own strong opinions, particularly of physicians' views of CAM, noting both a range in views but also how these might be shifting towards greater acceptance:

I think even physicians are recognising it as well. I don't mean 'even physicians' in a patronising way, but I think there is a move towards understanding that there's multiple forms of knowledge and multiple ways of knowing and thus multiple ways of healing. And that we do not want to throw the baby out with the bath water and reject everything that allopathic medicine has to offer nor do we want to go whole-heartedly, you know, and support everything alternative therapies have to offer. We do want to see a consistent and well-thought-out integration between the two of them. And I think that's the direction we're moving into.

(Midwife)

Thus, we found a range of views towards CAM integration among and between physicians, nurses and midwives in line with the literature available in this area. However, it is not clear what the implications of the differing attitudes have on the behaviour of these health professionals – this issue, to which we now turn, reveals other important factors affecting mainstream professionals' behaviour.

What they do regarding CAM

A key theme that emerges from the literature focusing upon mainstream professionals *vis-à-vis* CAM is of the potential slippage between attitudes and behaviours (Hirschkorn and Bourgeault 2005). Mainstream professionals may portray a particular attitude but this may not be consistent with their behaviour – more often than not their behaviour is more circumscribed than are their attitudes. In light of this trend, it is imperative to not only examine what physicians, nurses and midwives think but also what they do (or at least based on our data what they say they do). We begin our discussion here with the interest these professionals expressed in seeking training in various CAM modalities. We then turn towards how they may or may not use these modalities in everyday practice and when they refer to CAM practitioners.

Pursuing CAM training

Deciding whether or not to pursue training in a particular CAM modality is a strong indication of a mainstream provider's support of CAM integration efforts. A variety of factors appear to influence whether training is or will be undertaken. Similar to the way that the existence of evidence for the modality or lack thereof affects these professionals' views, it also appears to affect their behaviour. For example, the level of evidence influenced some physicians' willingness to undertake training in some CAM modalities:

Q: Would you ever consider taking formal training?
A: Yeah, I'd consider it if I had more time. Yeah.
Q: And what particular areas would you look into if you had more time?
A: Um, it would be interesting to look into massage therapy. I might consider looking into acupuncture or acupressure . . .
Q: And what would be the reasons for specifically massage or acupuncture or acupressure?
A: Uh, well I think in terms of acupuncture I think there's some good research, good evidence supporting its use. . . . So I can see where that would be beneficial. It would be nice to be able to offer patients something beyond what I do in the conventional practice.

(Physician)

Q: Would you ever consider training in any modality?
A: Hmm. Perhaps in acupuncture. That might be one area that I might consider. But that's probably the only one.
Q: Is there any reason why acupuncture is of more interest than most?
A: I think it's because of its long history and there's a lot of evidence on the effectiveness in many areas so I would be more likely to take an interest in that.

(Physician)

One physician even situated his view of training in conventional medicine and training in a CAM practice at the same level:

> I haven't had any formal training in any of the complementary alternative treatments, nor have I got formal training in say prescribing Bramapril which is a prescribed medication. I've got training in prescribing medications and I treat the complementary alternative ones as medications . . . looking at the evidence for whether they work or not and try to figure out whether there's a . . . scientific basis for prescribing them.

(Physician)

This was consistent with the reasons given by a number of the nurses for deciding to seek training. This is illustrated via the quotes below, the first from a nurse regarding therapeutic touch and the second a nurse interested in herbal medicine:

> The reason I chose therapeutic touch is because there is quite a bit of literature and I think some good evidence. I mean I shouldn't say good evidence, the studies are flawed. But if we compare it to what is out there for medical evidence for medical practice, it's certainly equal to that.
>
> (Nurse)

> I would be interested in learning more information about herbal and naturopathic remedies, but I really, I would like to know, I'd like to see more consistent evidence on those so I would even be interested in participating in some research regarding that because I know there's not the same regulations on herbal remedies as there are on obviously medications at the current time. But yeah, I would be interested in learning a bit more about some of those things.
>
> (Nurse)

Beyond the more general issue of evidence for the particular modality, health care professionals also had pragmatic reasons to seek training. For example, one physician noted how:

> My motivation would be informational. I'd just want to see what the purported rationale is for the treatments and what the toxicities are. I would like to learn about what the potential interactions are between those and the things that I prescribe.
>
> (Physician)

One of the nurses noted how she was most comfortable with incorporating those modalities that were not harmful:

> There's certain ones that I've learned about and I know that they're not harmful and therefore I feel comfortable with.
>
> (Nurse)

Overall there was some interest in particular CAM modalities among all provider groups. Midwives, for example, expressed particular interest in herbal medicines, homeopathy, aromatherapy and massage therapy as these would be important complements to the practice of maternity care. Many of the nurses interviewed mentioned their training in therapeutic touch such that it was, as one nurse put it, almost considered part of traditional care:

> I've done a little bit of training I guess in therapeutic touch which actually I guess in nursing we consider almost more of our traditional practice than consider it being a complementary therapy.
>
> (Nurse)

While the modalities adopted were perceived as requiring some relevance for their practice, those that could be easily undertaken in a short period of time – such as a workshop – were found to be most popular:

> I have talked with all kinds of midwives about how they're practising and I think the majority of midwives are pretty overwhelmed by their workload and it's really hard to think of getting a lot of expertise in another area.
>
> (Midwife)

This latter quote parallels the quote by the physician above who noted that one of the barriers to his pursuing CAM training was quite simply time. Those modalities such as chiropractic and other forms of manipulation were seen to be much more involved and therefore not feasible for adoption and integration. For example, one midwife states:

> I aim to practise midwifery. And if I was a herbalist, I wouldn't aim to be a midwife. It's possible of course that those two things could co-exist. Why not? But I think that it's unreasonable to expect that a midwife would have anything other than sort of a passing knowledge of other therapies, and perhaps be able to identify when they might be useful to a client.
>
> (Midwife)

Using CAM and referring to CAM providers

Similar to its influence on pursuing training, the level of knowledge of a CAM modality was noted as an important factor influencing the variability in professionals' ability and willingness to practise a particular CAM modality or to refer to an appropriate provider:

> Midwives do use complementary therapies, and the ones that don't generally say it's because they don't know enough about them so they're a bit hesitant.
>
> (Midwife)

> You can only do the things that you're trained to do, and you can't do the things really that other people are licensed to do, but you have to know who does what so that if you think there's something that your client will benefit from that you make a referral to that person.
>
> (Midwife)

Some of the physicians interviewed also note that they have in the past referred patients to CAM providers, one of the main reasons for such a referral being to address a health problem from a variety of perspectives. For example, one physician explains:

> I've had patients who I'm sending to acupuncturists, massage therapists, Shiatsu . . . at the same time that I'm treating them with drugs and with physiotherapy. It depends on how serious the problem is. There are times when you, again you need all the help you can get and multiple modalities are required simultaneously with people who are really in trouble. And you don't sit around wondering what the best therapy is. They're all, used properly they are complementary to each other.
>
> (Physician)

Midwives in particular noted that they encourage referrals and in some cases self-administration of CAM therapies:

> I think most of the midwives in the area are either recommending that their clients see someone who is trained in that area of medicine or are encouraging their patients to use some form or other, whether it's really an in-depth use of it or more of a shallow use of the botanicals and other medicines.
>
> (Midwife)

The midwives expressed a sense of pragmatism in their employment of CAM modalities – that is, doing what worked whether it was conventional or complementary:

> I mean there [are] homeopathic remedies that are used for resuscitating a baby instead of bag and mask. There [are] remedies for haemorrhage. We actually don't use remedies for those. We actually rely on good old fashioned pharmaceuticals for postpartum haemorrhage. You know, we don't [use them in], acute emergencies . . . But in a labour where somebody is maybe stuck in dilation, we use them.
>
> (Midwife)

Further, as was previously noted above regarding the influence of medical specialty on attitudes towards CAM, some respondents stated that a particular specialty also influenced their ability to practise CAM. For example, a nurse who worked in a couple of different units over the years explains:

> [You] seldom see [CAM] in intensive care. I have [also] never seen anybody doing anything of that kind in haemodialysis . . . because haemodialysis is just a kind of out-patient thing. They come in for the dialysis and then they go home so there's not much time for doing this kind of thing with them.
>
> (Nurse)

Thus, a structural relationship involving enough contact time with patients seems critical to nurses' ability to practise a CAM modality. This is consistent with the argument presented earlier by one of our medical respondents that the more positive views of nurses *vis-à-vis* CAM (in comparison to physicians) was due to nurses being there with the patient and more in line with a patient's desire to seek an alternative.

Another influence on the behaviour of these three groups relates to the inter-professional status differential, which is heightened by gender differences. For example, one nurse states:

> I just think women are more open and I think that as nurses we provide a lot of care to our clients particularly, and the way I was trained in the '60s and that kind of thing, there was a lot more touch. Like back rubs every day and a lot more time to sit and hold hands and that kind of thing. I think that's a shame that that's not there any more because I think it's a very healing thing.
>
> (Nurse)

Nurses and midwives were more likely than physicians to mention holism, caring or patient advocacy – whatever the source, these status differentials mean that in practice physicians' opinions tend to be more influential:

> I wouldn't want to step over any lines and be suggesting things that would upset the boat. You know, I don't want them going back to their doctor and saying, you know, some nurse suggested that they go do something weird. I'm very careful about that.
>
> (Nurse)

This situation was particularly exacerbated in the hospital setting. Other nurses and midwives indicated that although they might continue to use a particular form of CAM, they may not chart it, thus avoiding any confrontation. But in some cases, professionals have noted a change in the climate or have decided to openly use CAM even in the face of the negative reaction by physicians:

> Flaky to who, because 85 per cent of the population is interested in them and has used them at one time or another. So flaky in the eyes of the doctor? Well, we're kind of used to that, you know. That's not going to stop me.
>
> (Midwife)

The status of the mainstream provider using CAM also apparently affects the kind of attention that the therapy receives:

> Say, for example, therapeutic touch. You know therapeutic touch, the medical people used to just ignore it, but now you know there's been a few studies done to try to refute it and they're only done because of the popularity of it . . . But you don't get the medical backlash to it until somebody feels threatened by that. As long as you can sort of say 'Oh well, that's just those silly nurses just doing that. Big deal', that's one thing. But when, you know, somebody is suffering and you can't help them and then this nurse comes in and waves her hands over the person and they settle down and feel better, that makes you look silly doesn't it?
>
> (Physician)

It is also important to note that the relative status of these providers is in flux – midwifery being an important case in point in terms of its recent move from the margins to the mainstream in Canada – and this in turn may influence the degree to which their practices *vis-à-vis* CAM are recognised and adopted. Indeed, some of the midwives note the difference between the midwives that practised prior to integration (which occurred roughly in the early to late 1990s in each province) and those midwives who came on board as part of a regulated health profession:

> The newer, the younger midwives, haven't had as much use of complementary therapies but if they're working or did work with somebody that did utilise them in their practice, then they tend to continue with that use albeit cautiously. The ones that didn't have a lot of experience with it say that they'd like to, and if they have a colleague that starts using something, then again they'll maybe try something. So there's, because we still have the majority of our midwives are from a previous population that were practising outside of regulation, I think we still have a lot of that complementary and alternative medicine use that was part of that practice. So it would be interesting [to see what happens] in five years' time.
>
> (Midwife)

Discussion

In sum, our qualitative study of physicians, nurses and midwives revealed variability in attitudes and behaviour regarding CAM both within and between professions. Our data also reveals discrepancies between professionals' views and actions regarding CAM integration and reveals shifting attitudes and behaviour over time.

First, with respect to internal professional differences in attitudes and behaviour, we did not find, as Tovey (1997) did, that medical specialists were less open to CAM modalities. Indeed, the oncologists interviewed were quite open towards patients' use of CAM in certain circumstances. What affected these practitioners' opinions was the relative successfulness of their own therapies for the conditions they were treating. This is consistent with previous findings regarding general practitioners and oncologists (Bourgeault 1996). Specifically, that physicians were much more open to patients using CAM when their prognosis with conventional medicine was poor. It is important to note, however, that unlike Tovey (1997), we did not survey across all medical specialities so we are not arguing that our findings are generalisable to specialists. Rather, our qualitative design allowed us to delve further into the reasons behind the variability identified in our participants' responses. The specialty differences that emerged within nursing could be seen as largely due to the altered structural relations with patients (discussed further below). Other internal professional differences for physicians, nurses and midwives were due to that naturally expected variation in personal views on a controversial topic.

Second, similar to the findings of other studies regarding differences in attitudes and behaviour between professions, our data reveals a hierarchy of openness towards CAM. Drawing this argument further, nursing could be seen as representing a 'middling' position between, on the one hand, physicians' relative incompatible philosophy of practice relative to CAM and, on the other hand, midwives' place in the division of labour sometimes seen as complementary/alternative.

Again, our qualitative design does not enable us to identify statistically significant differences, but rather it enables us to uncover the factors that differentially influenced what these health care professionals think and do. Further, a key strength of our study is that it is empirically comparative by design – the differences in our study have emerged from a common methodology and thereby cannot be attributed to differences in research design.

Some of the factors we uncovered are consistent with Tovey's (1997) and Adams' (2006) assertion of the affinity between nurses and midwives (respectively) and CAM. Such an affinity might be related to a gendered compatibility and the structural situation of these professions having more frequent opportunity to discuss experience of CAM with patients than that afforded to physicians. However, it remains that the influences of gender and work structure are overlapping and would need to be teased apart – if possible – in further research into CAM integration.

Third, similar to the existing literature on mainstream professionals and CAM, we found there were some discrepancies between supportive attitudes and actual behaviour, particularly among nurses and midwives. This is where a theoretically influenced understanding of the inter-professional relationships is most instructive. Specifically, the finding that some nurses and midwives feel the need to curb their enthusiasm for CAM modalities either directly in the presence of an unsupportive physician, or indirectly within the context of hospital policies is telling of the influence of medical dominance. These limits on nurses' and midwives' behaviour was less of an issue when their views were comparable to the negative or ambivalent views of physicians *vis-à-vis* CAM.

Finally, our data suggests that there has been a shift towards more open attitudes and behaviours among all three groups of health professionals regarding CAM. Indeed, what is implicit in all of our interviews is the important influence of time in shifting how physicians, nurses and midwives think about CAM and what they do regarding its practice and integration, even with regard to some of those who are more ambivalent. Although it is difficult for us to tell based on our methods how this might be distributed among the groups, it was nevertheless a particularly salient issue for the physicians, nurses and midwives from a wide variety of settings. It can be confidently said that the status quo is undergoing a dramatic shift – what is uncertain is where such a shift will ultimately take mainstream health care professionals and CAM.

Note

1 Given the small practitioner/educator communities encompassed by the two universities sampled and thus the challenges involved in anonymising the data, we have opted to remove any descriptors from the quotations other than 'nurse', 'midwife' and 'physician'. While the range of specialties and structural locations of the professionals was important for our sampling strategy and for obtaining a range of perspectives, we do not believe that exclusion of this information in the body of this chapter detracts from the arguments we are presenting here.

Acknowledgements

We would like to acknowledge funding from the Canadian Institutes of Health Research through a New Investigator Award to I. Bourgeault and through a Doctoral Fellowship to K. Hirschkorn.

References

Abbott, A. (1988) *The System of Professions: An Essay on the Division of Expert Labour.* Chicago, IL and London: University of Chicago Press.

Adams, J. (2000) General practitioners, complementary therapies and evidence-based medicine: the defence of clinical autonomy. *Complementary Therapies in Medicine* 8(4): 248–52.

Adams, J. (2004) Demarcating the medical/non-medical border: occupational boundary-work within GPs' accounts of their integrative practice. In Tovey, P., Easthope, G. and Adams, J. (eds) *The Mainstreaming of Complementary and Alternative Medicine: Studies in Social Context.* London and New York: Routledge, pp. 140–57.

Adams, J. (2006) An exploratory study of complementary and alternative medicine in hospital midwifery: models of care and professional struggle. *Complementary Therapies in Clinical Practice* 12(1): 40–7.

Adams, J. and Tovey, P. (2001) Nurses' use of professional distancing in the appropriation of CAM: a text analysis. *Complementary Therapies in Medicine* 9(3): 136–40.

Allaire, A. D., Moos, M. K. et al. (2000) Complementary and alternative medicine in pregnancy: a survey of North Carolina certified nurse-midwives. *Obstetrics & Gynecology* 95(1): 19–23.

Astin, J. A., Marie, A. et al. (1998) A review of the incorporation of complementary and alternative medicine by mainstream physicians. *Archives of Internal Medicine* 158(21): 2303–10.

Baugniet, J., Boon, H. et al. (2000) Complementary/alternative medicine: comparing the view of medical students with students in other health care professions. *Family Medicine* 32(3): 178–84.

Berman, B. M., Bausell, R. B. et al. (1999) Compliance with requests for complementary-alternative medicine referrals: a survey of primary care physicians. *Integrative Medicine* 2(1): 11–17.

Berman, B. M., Bausell, R. B. et al. (2002) Use and referral patterns for 22 complementary and alternative medical therapies by members of the American College of Rheumatology: results of a national survey. *Archives of Internal Medicine* 162(7): 766–70.

Berman, B. M., Singh, B. B. et al. (1998) Primary care physicians and complementary-alternative medicine: training, attitudes, and practice patterns. *Journal of the American Board of Family Practice* 11(4): 272–81.

Bernstein, J. H. and Shuval, J. T. (1997) Nonconventional medicine in Israel: consultation patterns of the Israeli population and attitudes of primary care physicians. *Social Science & Medicine* 44(9): 1341–8.

Borkan, J., Neher, J. O. et al. (1994) Referrals for alternative therapies. *The Journal of Family Practice* 39(6): 545–50.

Botting, D. A. and Cook, R. (2000) Complementary medicine: knowledge, use and attitudes of doctors. *Complementary Therapies in Nursing & Midwifery* 6(1): 41–7.

Bourgeault, I. L. (1996) Physicians' attitudes toward patients' use of alternative cancer therapies. *CMAJ* 155(12): 1679–85.

Burg, M. A., Kosch, S. G. et al. (1998) Personal use of alternative medicine therapies by health science center faculty. *JAMA* 280(18): 1563.

Burns, E. and Blamey, C. (1994) Complementary medicine: using aromatherapy in
childbirth. *Nursing Times* 90(9): 54–60.

Burns, E., Blamey, C. et al. (2000a) The use of aromatherapy in intrapartum
midwifery practice: an observational study. *Complementary Therapies in Nursing
& Midwifery* 6(1): 33–4.

Burns, E., Blamey, C. et al. (2000b) Aromatherapy in childbirth: an effective
approach to care. *British Journal of Midwifery* 8(10): 639–43.

Cattell, E. (1999) Nurse practitioners' role in complementary and alternative medicine: active or passive? *Nursing Forum* 34(3): 14–23.

Chen, B., Bernard, A. et al. (1999) Differences between family physicians and
patients in their knowledge and attitudes regarding traditional Chinese medicine.
Integrative Medicine 2(2/3): 45–55.

Cohen, M. H. and Eisenberg, D. M. (2002) Potential physician malpractice liability
associated with complementary and integrative medical therapies. *Annals of
Internal Medicine* 136(8): 596–603.

Curry, A. and Smith, S. T. (1998) Information on alternative medicine: a collection
management issue. *Bulletin of the Medical Library Association* 86(1): 95–100.

DeKeyser, F. G., Cohen, B. B. et al. (2001) Knowledge levels and attitudes of staff
nurses in Israel towards complementary and alternative medicine. *Journal of
Advanced Nursing* 36(1): 41–8.

Dimond, B. (1998) Complementary medicine and midwifery practice *Practising
Midwife* 1(4): 12–13.

Eisenberg, D. M., Davis, R. B. et al. (1998) Trends in alternative medicine use in the
United States, 1990–1997: results of a follow-up national survey. *JAMA* 280(18):
1569–75.

Fitch, M. I., Gray, R. E. et al. (1999) Nurses' perspectives on unconventional
therapies. *Cancer Nursing* 22(3): 238–45.

Freidson, E. (1970) *Professional Dominance: The Social Structure of Medical Care.*
Chicago, IL: Aldine Publishing Company/Atherton Press.

Frisch, N. C. (2001a) Standards for holistic nursing practice: a way to think about
our care that includes complementary and alternative modalities. *Online Journal
of Issues in Nursing* 6(2): 4.

Frisch, N. C. (2001b) Nursing as a context for alternative/complementary modalities.
Online Journal of Issues in Nursing 6(2): Manuscript 2.

Glaus, A. (1988) The position of nursing: between school medicine and alternative
medicine. *Cancer Nursing* 11(4): 250–3.

Goldner, M. (2000) Integrative medicine: issues to consider in this emerging form of
health care. *Research in the Sociology of Health Care* (17): 215–36.

Goldszmidt, M., Levitt, C. et al. (1995) Complementary health care services: a
survey of general practitioner's views. *CMAJ* 153(1): 29–35.

Gray, R. E., Fitch, M. et al. (1998) A comparison of physician and patient perspectives on unconventional cancer therapies. *Psycho-Oncology* 7(6): 445–52.

Hasan, M. Y., Das, M. et al. (2000) Alternative medicine and the medical profession: views of medical students and general practitioners. *Eastern Mediterranean
Health Journal* 6(1): 25–33.

Hirschkorn, K. and Bourgeault, I. (2005) Conceptualizing mainstream health care providers' behaviours in relation to complementary and alternative medicine. *Social Science & Medicine* 61(1): 157–70.

Johnson, G. (2000) Should nurses practise complementary therapies? *Complementary Therapies in Nursing & Midwifery* 6(3): 120–3.

King, M. O. B., Pettigrew, A. C. et al. (1999) Complementary, alternative, integrative: have nurses kept pace with their clients? *Medsurg Nursing* 8(4): 249–57.

Lorenzo, P. (2003) Complementary therapies – they're not without risk. *RN* 66(1): 65–6, 68.

Mayer, C., Orr, S. et al. (2001) Alternative views . . . complementary therapies can work well alongside conventional nursing practice. *Nursing Standard* 15(16): 27.

Montbriand, M. J. (2000) Alternative therapies: health professionals' attitudes *Canadian Nurse* 96(3): 22–6.

Raisler, J. (2000) Midwifery care research: what questions are being asked? What lessons have been learned? *Journal of Midwifery & Women's Health* 45(1): 20–36.

Rose, S. (1994) Advantages of antenatal and postnatal aromatherapy. *British Journal of Midwifery* 2(3): 133–4.

Sakala, C. (1988) Content of care by independent midwives: assistance with pain in labor and birth. *Social Science & Medicine* 26(11): 1141–58.

Saks, M. (1996) From quackery to complementary medicine: the shifting boundaries between orthodox and unorthodox medical knowledge. In Cant, S. and Sharma, U. (eds) *Complementary and Alternative Medicines: Knowledge in Practice*. London and New York: Free Association Books, pp. 27–43.

Saks, M. (2000) Professionalization, politics and CAM. In Kelner, M., Wellman, B., Pescosolido, B. and Saks, M. *Complementary and Alternative Medicine: Challenge and Change*. Australia: Harwood Academic Publishers. pp. 223–38.

Salmenpera, L., Suominen, T. et al. (1998) Oncology nurses' attitudes towards alternative medicine. *Psycho-Oncology* 7(6): 453–9.

Sharma, U. (2000) Medical pluralism and the future of CAM. In Kelner, M., Wellman, B., Pescosolido, B. and Saks, M. *Complementary and Alternative Medicine: Challenge and Change*. Australia: Harwood Academic Publishers, pp. 211–22.

Siahpush, M. (1999) A critical review of the sociology of alternative medicine: research on users, practitioners and the orthodoxy. *Health* 4(2): 159–78.

Silverman, R. (1995) Use of alternative therapies in childbirth. *British Journal of Midwifery* 3(4): 196–200.

Smith, M. (1991) Complementary support. *Nursing Times* 87(32): 36–8.

Straub, L. A. and Henley, E. (2000) Complementary medicine in rural Illinois: provider views. *Rural Research Report* 11(8): 1–8.

Strauss, A. and Corbin, J. (1990) *Basics of Qualitative Research: Grounded Theory Procedures and Techniques*. Newbury Park, CA: Sage.

Taylor, B. (2002) Becoming a reflective nurse or midwife: using complementary therapies while practising holistically. *Complementary Therapies in Nursing & Midwifery* 8: 62–8.

Tiran, D. (2003) Implementing complementary therapies into midwifery practice. *Complementary Therapies in Nursing & Midwifery* 9(1): 10–13.

Tiran, D. and Mack, S. (2000) *Complementary Therapies for Pregnancy and Childbirth*. Edinburgh: Bailliere Tindall.

Tovey, P. (1997) Contingent legitimacy: UK alternative practitioners and intersectoral acceptance. *Social Science & Medicine* 45(7): 1129–33.

Tovey, P. and Adams, J. (2001) 'Primary care as intersecting social worlds. *Social Science & Medicine* 52: 695–706.

Tovey, P. and Adams, J. (2002) Towards a sociology of CAM and nursing. *Complementary Therapies in Nursing & Midwifery* 8(1): 12–16.

Tovey, P. and Adams, J. (2003) Nostalgic and nostophobic referencing and the authentication of nurses' use of complementary therapies. *Social Science & Medicine* 56(7): 1469–80.

Trevelyan, J. (1996) A true complement? *Nursing Times* 92(5): 42–3.

Verhoef, M. J., Best, A. et al. (2002) Role of complementary medicine in medical education: opinions of medical educators. *Annals of the Royal College of Physicians and Surgeons of Canada* 35: 166–70.

Verhoef, M. J. and Sutherland, L. R. (1995a) General practitioners' assessment of and interest in alternative medicine in Canada. *Social Science & Medicine* 41(4): 511–15.

Verhoef, M. J. and Sutherland, L. R. (1995b) Alternative medicine and general practitioners: opinions and behaviour. *Canadian Family Physician* 41: 1005–11.

Wilkinson, J. M. and Simpson, M. D. (2002) Personal and professional use of complementary therapies by nurses in NSW, Australia. *Complementary Therapies in Nursing & Midwifery* 8: 142–7.

The emerging role of alternative midwifery within the wider socio-political sphere

A focus upon alternative birth care providers and their relationship with conventional medicine

Paaige K. Turner

Introduction

The growing use of complementary and alternative medicine (CAM) by patients and medical providers across late modern societies is increasing the narratives available for constructing the meanings of health, health care and the occupational and organisational roles of health care providers. Although it might be tempting to assume that the infusion of CAM practices into conventional medical settings will seed the growth of new models of health care and delivery, the fact is that many of these CAM practices are grounded in ontological and epistemological assumptions that differ and in some cases oppose the assumptions of biomedicine (Coulter 2004).

In this chapter, I provide a case study of the intersection of conventional and alternative birth care practices. Although research has focused on how conventional medical practices might be open to alternative practices (Conroy et al. 2000; Jonas 2002), it is also important to understand how operating within the dominant socio-political system might affect alternative practices and providers. This study provides one reading of the experiences of one group of birth care providers who, although embedded within current socio-political systems, seek to enact alternative definitions of birth, birth support and the role of birth care provider. The chapter focuses upon the emerging role of alternative birth care providers and their relationship with conventional medicine.

The intersection of CAM and conventional medicine

In the recent past, alternative forms of medicine were contained within the margins of medical care in the United States and other late modern societies. Today, however, patients, providers and even medical schools are demonstrating an increased interest in learning about and using CAM (Conroy et al. 2000; Kligler 1996; Moyad 2001) which has prompted a call to investigate how such practices and technologies can be integrated with conventional medicine in contemporary health care systems (White House Commission on Complementary and Alternative Medicine Policy 2002). This integration or intersection is particularly tenuous, given that conventional medicine and CAM have emerged from multiple paradigms that enjoy differing degrees of legitimacy and social centrality. Although these paradigmatic differences affect many practices, particularly relevant to the argument presented here are the relationships between the mind and body, the provider and the healing process, and determining appropriate evidence for establishing quality care.

First is the relationship of mind and body. Grosz (1994) has argued that the predominant ideology is the heir of Cartesian modes of reasoning, wherein the mind and body are separate entities, and that the body exists as a tool that is animated by an acting subjectivity and/or as a vehicle for expression of that subjectivity. Subsequently, for conventional medicine, the body exists as a biological, metaphysical reality that is reducible to its separate components and is the primary focus of treatment. 'In the first line of investigation, the body is primarily regarded as an object for the natural sciences, particularly for the life sciences, biology and medicine' (Grosz 1994: 8). CAM, however, often conceptualises the mind/body as integrated or does not even make a distinction between mind and body – the body is a unique system that, by virtue of its design, has within its disposal all that it needs to achieve a state of health (Davis-Floyd 1990; Mitford 1992).

Second is the relationship of the provider to the process of healing. The instantiation of the scientific method as the dominant epistemology and separation of the subject/object supports the assumption of objectivism that divides the one who looks and the one looked on (Thackray 1980). In conventional medicine, the doctor is placed at the centre of the healing act. The doctor conducts an examination, makes a diagnosis and determines a course of treatment. In CAM, the provider might serve more as a guide who helps patients to monitor their own bodies and determine their individual health goals (Coulter 2004) – the practitioner and the patient mutually and reciprocally determine a course of treatment. This places the provider as peripheral and the relationship as central to the healing process. CAM providers often prefer to develop an ongoing relationship with patients by seeing them when they are free of symptoms to help the individual sustain a continual state of health (Reed et al. 2000).

Underlying these issues is what will count as both quality and evidence of quality. Quality is a highly ambiguous construct within health care, particularly depending on whether it modifies care or life (Donabedian 1980):

There are many approaches to defining quality, including: (1) a transcendent approach where quality is undefined but evident when it exists; (2) a product-based approach where the product is measured by the quantity of its component attributes; (3) a user-based approach where the measure of quality is its ability to satisfy the customer; (4) a manufacturing-based approach where quality is conformance to standards; and (5) a value-based approach where quality is excellence at an affordable price.

(Stichler and Weiss 2001: 59–60)

Many of these definitions emerged out of a combination of specific historical events that also ground conventional medicine. For example, the instantiation of the scientific method as the dominant epistemology defined a specific type of data as appropriate (Thackray 1980), and rapid increases in technology provided the technical tools for gathering and assessing this type of data (Pursell 1980). Subsequently, conventional medicine tends to rely on epidemiological and outcome measures, such as utilisation patterns, mortality rates, clinical trials, compliance with medical association guidelines and regulations, and appropriate accreditation (Colton 2000; Frohock 2002). CAM approaches tend to invoke a more transcendental approach when determining what will count as evidence of quality (Jonas 2002). For individuals adhering to a CAM approach, a quality outcome does not necessarily imply the elimination of the health concern. Instead, such a quality outcome might be defined as the integration of the health issue with regard to the individual's wider lifeworld or assisting the individual with emotional issues.

It is clear that both conventional and CAM definitions of health and health practices are embedded within ideologies that are neither natural nor neutral. Rather, they have emerged out of and are sustained by specific historical events and discursive practices that have led to the predominance of one over another (Ehrenreich and English 1973; Foucault 1973). Subsequently, individuals who practise alternative forms of health care operate as a cognitive minority

whose view of the world differs significantly from the one generally taken for granted in their society . . . The status of a cognitive minority is thus invariably an uncomfortable one – not necessarily because the majority is repressive or intolerant, but simply because it refuses to accept the minority's definitions for reality yes as 'knowledge'.

(Berger 1969: 6–7; original emphasis)

As alternative health care providers (including alternative birth care providers) move into the current medical system they must negotiate their ideological differences regarding the relation of the mind and body, the relationship of the provider to the process of healing, and what will count as both quality and evidence of quality as a cognitive minority whose knowledge is suspect. Future definitions of health, birth care and midwifery will depend on how that intersection is negotiated.

Paradox cycles second level

Although the intersection of conventional birth care and midwifery can be understood as a potential site for integration, assimilation, or contradiction, in this chapter I focus on contradiction to highlight those meanings that will require the most amount of negotiation and, therefore, a greater potential for influencing constructions of midwifery. Indeed, Conquergood (1991) has argued for the need to focus on discourse at the borderlands or busy intersections because 'meaning is contested and struggled for in the interstices, *in between* structures' (p. 184; original emphasis). Thus, I align myself with researchers who view contradiction and inconsistency not as problems to be solved but as moments of meaning creation (Chesebro 1984).

According to Wood and Conrad (1983) a paradox requires that three injunctions merge: a primary negative injunction which prohibits a particular action through a threat to withhold rewards or deliver punishments; a secondary injunction that is inconsistent with the primary; and a tertiary injunction that prohibits the person with less power from leaving the field either psychologically or physically.

Paradoxes do not, however, exist in isolation from other systems of meaning. Informed by postmodernist thought (Lyotard 1991) it is possible to approach paradox as an interaction cycle or web. For a postmodernist, it is not possible to operate outside a system of meaning, and which system of meaning is constructed as 'real' is an issue of power. Thus, the response of the person with less power might not perpetuate the initial paradox, but it might perpetuate an alternative paradox that sustains the broader 'macro-paradox' (Wendt 1998: 333) or, in this instance, the predominant ideology and medical practices. It is particularly important, therefore, to broaden analysis and to attend to not just the paradox but also to the response and its relationship to the larger world (in the case of alternative birth care this can relate to the relationship of CAM practices and underlying assumptions to those of conventional medicines among other issues).

Embedded within a paradox cycle is power: to define behaviour, to keep the interaction in play, or to validate an appropriate response. It is not an authoritative power, which demands compliance; rather, it is power that emerges and exists within the relation of meanings. Thus, this project conceptualises power as 'the multiplicity of force relations immanent in the sphere in which they operate and which constitute their own organization'

(Foucault 1990: 92). By doing so, the actions of alternative midwives are situated within the larger socio-political sphere to articulate the emergent meanings and their implications for defining midwifery within a broader inter-professional context.

Methods

In order to highlight my arguments further this chapter will focus upon field-work conducted at a birth centre located at a Midwestern city in the USA. This centre was founded in 1993 and at the time of the study was the only freestanding birth centre in the state. In this research, I employed an embodied, interpretive interactionist methodology to focus on 'the point of view that confers meaning on problematic symbolic interaction' (Denzin 2001: 32) – moments in which individuals define themselves and relations to each other.

The women I engaged were either certified nurse-midwives (CNMs) or non-licenced, apprentice-trained midwives operating under the supervision of the CNMs providing midwifery care at the birth centre. To achieve robust and full-bodied qualitative research (Sandelowski 2002), multiple forms of data, including documents, interviews and field notes were collected via participative observation over a four-month period. This allowed meanings to be nested providing a robust representation of the play of meaning at the intersection of conventional and CAM practices. My procedures for data collection (including means for ensuring confidentiality), storage and analysis were approved by the appropriate institutional review board and included the following means for ensuring confidentiality of the participants.

Throughout the research process, I fed back my thoughts, confusions and, finally, my writings to the women who participated. In addition, I shared my ideas with midwives in other states and published part of my reflections in a midwifery magazine. In all cases, the women enthusiastically validated that the issues of name, work, licensing and technology were central to their experiences operating with the dominant socio-political system.

Analysis: living at the intersection

Claiming the name

'We are the guardians of the normal process' (Laura). The denotative meaning of midwife is 'to be with woman'. What midwives say midwifery is provides insight into what midwives want to be and what they think they should be, thus revealing/creating/responding to systems of beliefs. More-over, what they say midwifery is not also provides insight.

Midwifery is . . .

When directly asked what midwifery is, overwhelmingly, midwives drew on the following reoccurring concepts. Midwifery is (a) a philosophy based on the (b) normalcy and naturalness of pregnancy and labour (c) that helps women accept responsibility for their decisions (d) by establishing an ongoing relationship, and (e) to be with woman.

> Well, the quote definition of midwifery care is the independent care of essentially *normal, healthy women* through their childbearing years and beyond. But probably on a more personal level, what is midwifery care? I think it means *with women*. And I think it's [an] incredibly unusual *relationship that gets established* between a woman giving birth and the caregiver. It's, I don't know, it's part of being, a part of a growth, part of *assisting a couple* to kind of grow through a growth period *of accepting a lot of personal responsibility* and helping them make decisions about their own care. I'm kind of wandering.
>
> (Pam; emphasis added)

These beliefs resonated in the physical space and practices as well. The Birth Centre was a house complete with a swing set on the right lawn. The kitchen had a hot tub for labouring in the breakfast nook as well as food supplies that any individual could prepare without permission. In the living room were couches, books and bulletin boards that had articles pinned to them about water births, episiotomy rates and epidurals. In the dining room, there were computers and desks, as well as clients' records. The midwives told clients that they had access to their medical records at all times and that they were responsible for conducting and recording some of the basic assessments (e.g. urine tests).

Midwifery is not . . .

Derrida (1982) argues that a sign's meaning is inscribed in a system of *différance*, where signs both differ from and defer each other. When one signifier is invoked it differs from all other signifiers. For example, we understand the meaning of white because it differs from black, cat, snow, etc. In addition, signifiers temporally defer all other signs. For example, to invoke white is to not invoke black, cat, snow, etc. at this time. Those meanings are set aside. Thus, the meaning of any one sign is linked to the meanings of those it differs from and defers. Subsequently, what is identified as not midwifery simultaneously constitutes what is midwifery. When describing what a midwife is not or what a midwife does not do, the informants repeatedly positioned themselves in opposition to doctors, hospitals, or technology as sanctioned by the scientific paradigm:

LAURA: I mean an OB can do probably more of the things than I can count that we, you know, learn to do, than we can do, you know, are allowed to do. Like caesareans, using forceps, all these sort of technical things that they have higher training for.

INTERVIEWER: You don't use forceps?

LAURA: No. No. That's a *doctor thing*.

Where alternative birthing supplies (e.g. hot tub) were displayed openly, conventional birthing supplies (e.g. gauze, foetal monitoring devices) were hidden in armoires or cabinets. This simultaneous claiming and denying of specific practices as midwifery creates a potential point of intersection and paradox. First, midwives claim to be attendants at normal births, to follow a philosophy based on the normalcy of pregnancy and labour. However, they also are differentiated from a physician, do not use 'doctor thing' technology, and are different from the conventional medical care model, and yet the predominant ideology of birth is based on a model wherein physicians deliver babies using 'doctor thing' technology (Gélis 1991). A quick survey of births on The Learning Channel's *Maternity Ward* and narratives told by women about what they anticipate birth will be like (Pollock 1999) substantiate this with themes of women hooked to numerous apparatuses while doctors manage their labour. Thus, a potential paradox emerges wherein a midwife is not a physician (primary injunction prohibiting action) but a physician is the person who delivers babies (secondary injunction inconsistent with primary injunction). The midwife must then face the challenge of defining herself or himself as one who delivers babies and yet is not a physician. Alternatively she or he must redefine her or his midwifery to align with the predominate ideology.

Legal definitions of midwifery

The legal system provides another venue for defining midwifery. In this locality, the state code considers a person who practises midwifery without a licence to have committed a class D felony.[1] At a different point, however, the state code refers to a statute making a person who practises medicine without a licence guilty of a misdemeanour. Thus, an individual can face sanctions by the Medical Licensing Board, a misdemeanour charge, or a class D felony charge depending on her or his status (nurse-midwife vs lay midwife) and the charge brought against her or him (practising without a licence vs practising midwifery). The only basis for differentiating which statute applies is the name of the provider and type of licence, not the type of behaviour or quality of treatment. Indeed, Pam recognised this contradiction when she commented that there are bad obstetricians and bad midwives out there; licensing did not guarantee what type of treatment you got. She, however, chose to be licensed to provide her clients with a statement about who she was and obtain the needed physician backup. It is this need to have backup that prohibits midwives from leaving the field if they wish to operate within the dominant socio-political system (tertiary injunction).

The combination of the primary, secondary and tertiary injunctions creates some potential challenges and opportunities for midwives. When midwives are defined as not physicians, the possibility for midwives to be constructed as 'other' to provide physicians with their own subjectivity is increased. Similarly to de Beauvoir's (1961) argument that men are constructed as subjects via their construction of women as 'other', midwives might become the 'other' that defines physicians as the standard provider of labour support and care. This might have the effect of keeping midwives on the margin and defining their work as CAM, thereby limiting both their participation and their influence in the socio-political system. Alternatively, by defining themselves as different from a physician, they resist efforts to make them like a physician, sustaining their system of meaning about birth and enhancing the potential that their beliefs might endure and influence conventional beliefs about the role of labour support and care. The claiming-the-name paradox becomes a potential intersection for defining who is a midwife both internally and externally. Moreover, it nests within the need to operate as a recognised occupational category.

Is it work?

To claim the name of midwife is to claim an occupation, thereby requiring that one's activities be situated in some manner within the larger economic system. The midwives at the Birth Centre draw on many of the same concepts (e.g. pay, duration, intensity, training and location) that Clair (1996) found determined what counts as a real job. These concepts are consistent with capitalism's definition of work (Smith 1776/1937).

> And I think it has to do with the *kind of hours* you keep . . . So I think that's what *makes it work* . . . And plus, it's *intense* responsibility. But then the minute there is the time when you need to be, like, on your toes, and you know, really basically assessing, you know, or assuring that this mother and this baby are gonna stay healthy and alive, you know, I mean it really is life and death. *That's when it feels like work* . . . Not kind of, but it does, so that's, that's what, so it is work in the, if you look at it at what the job is as a whole. So, I *call it work.*
> (Laura)

Laura vacillates between situations in which she does consider her activities as work and ones in which she does not. However, the midwives also rejected capitalistic definitions of work by using qualifiers or alternative labels, such as 'the good work' or 'what I am'.

JULIE: I think, to me it's a gift that I share. And I get paid for it. And see, I did it for many years for no pay.

TRUDY: Well, I get paid for it [laughs]. But I do not consider it . . . Because I like coming to work.

Given the predominance of capitalistic constructions of work, rejecting the definition of midwifery as work might result in perceptions that midwives are less legitimate than conventional medical occupations and that they should be paid less or not at all. Indeed, during several conversations, the midwives mentioned that women would call them and expect them to provide care at a reduced rate or even for free if they did not have insurance. These women clearly felt that defining midwifery within only one realm created a tension for them. They expressed concern about their inability to offer their services for a reduced rate given that many of the women who made the request were using public forms of health insurance and could not afford to pay for the type of 'with woman' care (the definition of midwifery) the centre offers. Thus, the midwives become trapped in a paradox that says Work is X, Y and Z only (primary injunction); midwifery is X, Y, Z and A, B (secondary injunction) and sometimes only some of these. Finally, their need to receive insurance payments and desire to help women keeps them within the dominant field (tertiary injunction). Thus, their efforts to resist the claiming-the-name paradox by distancing themselves from physicians and retaining their focus upon being 'with woman' might invoke the work paradox where being 'with woman' is not work. The need to negotiate both of these in order to obtain insurance effectively creates a double bind.

Getting a licence, demonstrating quality

Licensing is a means for ensuring that individuals who identify as members of an occupational category have met specific qualifications. It simultaneously allows individuals to assess the qualifications of health care practitioners, provides a means of monitoring those practitioners and is a public performance of legitimisation and protection that must be negotiated continually.

A licence provides the possibility of operating within the legal system and of obtaining malpractice insurance, insurance payment for services, obstetrical back-up, access to medications, hospital privileges and recourse for non-payment of debts. In short, with the licence comes the promise of protection and acceptance by the medical and business communities. In the health care industry, quality assurance can mean the difference between life and death. Quality health care of any kind must sustain the life and health of the individuals involved and thus can become intricately linked with safety. As such, the staff at the Birth Centre were quite rightly concerned with maintaining and documenting safe procedures designed to protect their patients as well as to maintain their licence.

The interesting question that was not discussed explicitly by them or asked by me was, 'What is quality?' Instead, discussions about quality often focused on how to provide quality midwifery care while meeting the licensing requirements. Birth Centre staff members agreed that by providing yearly reports, the external requirements for quality guidelines would be met. However, these reports, which are also provided to prospective clients, include statistics about average age of mothers, length of labours, biggest baby, smallest baby, transfer rates for mothers and babies, caesarean section rates and episiotomy rates. These statistical representations of medical outcomes are grounded in the conventional biomedical model and focus on measurable, rational definitions. In contrast, when the midwives participating in the study discussed the meaning of midwifery the issues raised included nurturing, being part of growth, helping couples take personal responsibility, making clients feel safe and comfortable, helping in general and keeping track of practices. One non-licensed, apprentice-trained midwife stated,

> The important part that makes midwifery different is the philosophy that focuses on things that aren't quantifiable. The, you know, what she did last week with her kids and how that's affecting her pregnancy.
> (Eliza)

In many ways, the Birth Centre staff are required to talk in terms of the medical model in order to refute its claims of lower safety and lax procedures in birth centres. By doing so, the midwives are talking in a language with which physicians, nurses, and their clients are familiar. Moreover, it is doubtful if reports about client satisfaction, growth and responsibility would satisfy the health department's requirement for 'quality assurance guidelines'. Nevertheless, the staff did not feel that this was a problem. Rather, they were upset that even when they spoke in the discourse of conventional medical providers, they were still ignored or minimised. They often talked about how members of the conventional medical community ignored studies conducted by their own colleagues that showed birth centre and home births to be as safe as, if not safer than, hospital births. During my interviews and public tours, they pointed to academic articles posted in the living room that articulated the advantages of midwifery and the risks of conventional care (e.g. failure rates of epidurals and comparison of C-section rates across the world). Scott's (1990) concept of public transcripts and hidden transcripts provides a potential way of understanding why, even though midwives were using evidence appropriate to the conventional paradigm, they felt silenced. Scott argues that although the public transcript might be congruent with the demands of those in power, the dominant might suspect that it is only a performance, thus discounting its authenticity. 'It is but a short step from such skepticism to the view, common among many dominant groups, that those beneath them are deceitful, shamming, and lying by nature' (Scott 1990: 3).

If the conventional medical community doubts the goals of the midwives, even when their information conforms to conventional standards of evidence and supports the medical community's goals, the midwives' information might be discounted or constructed as inaccurate. Thus, midwives cannot use conventional medical care providers' discourse of quality (primary injunction), yet they must establish their quality based on what counts as quality in conventional medical practices (secondary injunction). Finally, the paradox is completed by a tertiary injunction that prevents them from leaving the field of meaning. Recall, midwives' abilities to achieve recognition by using the discourse of the dominant paradigm while still operating from an alternative paradigm might be limited by the construction of them as a cognitive minority whose assumptions differ significantly from those generally accepted within the specific locality. Subsequently they cannot, in effect, leave the field of meaning that has ascribed them as a cognitive minority, nor may they leave the field of meaning around what will count as quality or evidence of quality for licensing.

To use or not to use technology

Access to, and the defining of, technology has historically been a moment of potential meaning negotiation. In midwifery, differing systems of meaning play within each other, denoting who should have access to technology, what will constitute an appropriate response, and what will count as technology.

Access to technology

A question exists concerning who should have access to technology. A primary injunction can be identified that constrains midwives' use of technology: The midwife is not a physician (recall the naming paradox) and may not use certain forms of technology that have been sanctioned by the scientific paradigm (i.e. doctor thing technology) including forceps and vacuum extractors, or order epidurals or caesarean sections. However, a secondary injunction is also in play that says technology is necessary to have a safe delivery and be a competent care giver. This paradox is not new. During the early 1900s, doctors condemned midwives for maternal deaths and infant blindness while denying them access to anti-haemorrhaging medications and silver nitrate (Varney 1987).

Responses to technology paradoxes

The women I spoke with predominantly referred to technology to differentiate how a midwife handles events compared to conventional providers (name paradox) or as an example of interaction between the midwife and the conventional medical community. Responses to paradoxes that surround technology included acknowledging the paradox only in certain situations (Putnam 1983) and reframing the paradox so that it does not apply (Wood and Conrad 1983).

The first type of response was acknowledgement within certain situations. Women do need to have technology to have a safe birth, but only in high-risk situations. After stating that forceps (and other forms of technology) were a 'doctor thing', Laura noted that these were sometimes necessary:

> But there are sick women who get pregnant. You know insulin dependent diabetics, or people with heart problems, you know there's a lot of stuff. And that to me seems like obstetrics.
>
> (Laura)

The second type of response reframed the situation so that the paradox did not apply (Wood and Conrad 1983). Technology was recast as the cause of problems not the solution:

> I think the medical establishment has medicalised birth so much, they don't consider different mindsets. I think the medical establishment has medicalised birth so much, they don't consider it safe until afterwards, the baby's come out and it's OK. And so therefore they intervene even in normal labours. And intervening in normal labours can cause a lot of problems, a lot of potential problems.
>
> (Pam)

Pam's statement simultaneously recasts technology as the cause of the problem and resists efforts to define normal childbirth as needing interventions (e.g. forceps). Moreover, she casts the intervention as that which makes the birth not normal. Thus, the paradox is recast such that the primary injunction becomes the notion that women should experience a normal childbirth with a secondary injunction, women should not use technology. This is similar to what Clair et al. (1993) have termed 'alternaturing' – it not only reframes or recasts the paradox but also transforms what was once considered normal to expose and educate people about the paradox.

Defining what will count as technology

Another effort to reframe the technology paradox creates two categories of technology: hierarchical (midwifery) and dichotomous (conventional birth care providers). The midwives I spoke with talked in terms of a scale of low-tech and high-tech interventions. Under the rubric of midwifery, technology can be used on an as-needed basis, moving gradually up a hierarchy from offering a drink of water to amnio infusion. In contrast, midwives perceive the conventional medical community as jumping from no intervention to complete intervention, suggesting a dichotomous view of technology.

One way in which the midwives sustained this perspective was in the recurrent telling of the story here titled 'The Cycle of Interventions or Complications'. Three midwives told this story in a very similar manner. First, you (a labouring woman) arrive at the hospital too early, but they admit you anyway. After you have been there a while, they check and find you're only a few centimetres (because you were not really in labour yet), so they give you Pitocin, which requires that they hook you up to a monitor and that you lie flat on your back. Because you are flat on your back, you cannot get up and move, so the pain is increased and you are given an epidural. The epidural diminishes your ability to push, and the monitor often shows the baby in distress when it is only momentary. Because the baby is in distress, you wind up with a C-section – all because you were not really in labour when you were admitted. Although the story has a progressive structure (first, second, third), it is told as a package (this is what you might/will wind up with if you go to a hospital with an obstetrician), thus dichotomising the use of technology.

Midwives discursively create a hierarchy of technology and achieve two things. First, they construct a place wherein they can use technology while still sustaining their beliefs in no or low intervention (e.g. low-tech methods). Second, they can provide the entire scale of technology to their clients (from drink to amnio infusion via their back-up obstetrician). Because they portray the conventional medical community as having a dichotomous view, doctors can provide only no intervention or the cycle of complications. Thus, the technology paradox becomes redefined such that midwives discursively offer you a broader range of technology. Recurrent phrases, in which the midwives told clients that they could 'offer them more' (e.g. tubs, continual support, lower episiotomy rates), also reflect this attitude that with a midwife, a person has more choices, not fewer. Moreover, the redefining of the paradox alters the original premise. Now, birth care providers (midwife or doctor) can use technology (as redefined in the midwives' discourse), and a really good birth care provider would offer a range of technology. Doctors do not; therefore, they are not really good birth care providers. The paradox is turned back on itself in an attempt to alter the nature of the original paradox.

Moving through webs of meaning

Although this chapter has so far presented individual paradoxes separately, it was also clear from the analysis that all of the paradoxes could become relevant in a single moment and combine in ways that could challenge an alternative birth care provider's ability to negotiate her or his beliefs and practices with conventional beliefs and practices. For example, one midwife (Maddie) expressed concerns that birth care providers need to check in (literally and figuratively) more because they did not have or want to have the technology that would allow them to decrease personal monitoring:

> Blood pressures after the birth is another example. No one does them. They don't do them the way they're supposed to be done. You know, in the hospital, what they do is they slap the cuff on your arm, and they turn the machine on to do those blood pressures every fifteen minutes for the first hour. And this machine takes care of it. You know, we wouldn't do that here. Then we're asking these birth assistants to, as well as doing everything else, they're supposed to do the blood pressures every fifteen minutes for the first hour. So when I get these charts and I go, 'OK. You have to do this every fifteen minutes for the first hour.' Well, you know, I get this, 'she was breast-feeding'.
>
> (Maddie)

Maddie later talked about how taking blood pressures is a means of ensuring that the mother is stable and also a way of ensuring that the Centre retained its accreditation. Once again, the intersection of alternative and conventional weaves a potentially contradictory system of meaning. First, to exist, the Birth Centre needs to make money. Making money requires that its employees' activities be defined as work and not as a gift (work paradox). The Centre needs to be licensed to receive insurance payments (licensing paradox). To be licensed, they must meet quality standards (quality paradox) that are defined according to measurable, observable statistics consistent with the beliefs of conventional medicine, not necessarily according to the goals of midwifery (claiming-the-name paradox), so they strive to demonstrate quality according to conventional definitions while 'doing everything else'. Furthermore, the use of a blood pressure cuff would solve the licensing paradox yet invokes the paradox regarding normal birth not using technology (technology paradox). Thus, the response to one paradox might weave to another.

Implications for mainstreaming alternative medicine

Overall, this study suggests that as conventional and alternative approaches to (birth) health care intersect, it is important to attend to the implications for CAM practices and providers. Specifically, we need to provide continuous monitoring if we are bringing CAM into the mainstream, bringing the mainstream into CAM, or some combination therein. Although this study is limited in scope to a specific group of alternative birth care providers, it suggests that we need to be particularly conscious of the following issues and their implications not only for the practice of CAM but also for the system of beliefs that sustain those practices.

First, we need to be conscious of the power of naming. Currently, midwives' legitimacy is closely tied to their training and licensing established by conventional health care standards. The inclusion of midwives (and, more recently, doulas) in conventional birth care settings might serve to define them in relation to physicians, using pre-existing conceptualisations about what it means to be a birth care provider, rather than bring midwifery-type care into the mainstream. This might have the effect of redefining what it means to be a midwife in a manner that negates the reason it has been brought into the mainstream. A second issue is the complex relation of provider, patient and responsibility. This is a particularly sensitive and timely issue given the current insurance environment. Obstetricians, as well as other physicians, are experiencing significant problems obtaining affordable malpractice insurance, given that birth is constructed as high risk and that awards tend to be large in infant malpractice suits. The structure of insurance practices places the physician at the centre of the healing act and ascribes responsibility to her or him for a successful outcome. Midwives, however, operate from a paradigm of mutual responsibility that defines success not only in terms of outcome but also in terms of emotional and mental well-being. When midwives move into the mainstream, they must find a way to negotiate their belief in shared responsibility with their needs to define what they do as work, as a legitimate occupation, and obtain insurance coverage for both themselves and their patients.

In this study, the midwives identified several instances in which they expressed these paradoxes, yet there are also wider questions to be asked of such developments. For example, what if a patient turns down a medication, such as a vitamin K injection, a widespread practice in hospitals, and the child develops bleeding in his or her brain? Who is responsible? How can midwives be midwives and demonstrate competence when competence is currently defined by the use of standard practices 'consistent with professional knowledge' (Lohr 1990), when their standard practice is to allow individuals to make informed choices? Do midwives walk away from a client who will not do what they recommend to avoid being charged with malpractice or losing their licence? Although conventional medical providers also face similar challenges, their beliefs that the provider is at the centre of the healing act provide an alternative reference point for making decisions. However, if we continue to place providers at the centre of the healing act and separate them from the relationship, efforts to empower patients to make their own decisions will be limited by the current system of meaning. Indeed, the conventional paradigm will direct us to continue asking questions that will increasingly no longer make sense – such as 'Who is responsible for ensuring quality? The provider or the patient?' – rather than asking 'How do providers and patients ensure quality together?' This suggests that both providers and patients need to investigate how to broaden the concept of responsibility by moving beyond current conceptualisations of the relationship between provider and patient.

Third, operating within the dominant paradigm might serve to admit alternative providers into conventional medical settings yet might do little to change the status of those providers in two ways. The standards for quality and licensing are based on a different paradigm and alternative birth providers utilising CAM will never be able to comply fully and demonstrate quality according to the dominant definition. Thus, their practices will continue to appear and feel incomplete, patched together and, therefore, suspect. Moreover, even efforts to rationalise their practices using the discourse of the dominant paradigm might be viewed as merely a performance to participate in conventional settings. CAM might, therefore, be viewed as lacking evidence for establishing quality and alternative health care providers framed as lacking integrity. If midwives are ranked by name and their discourse discredited, they will continue to be pushed to the margin and constructed as low status in comparison to those whose discourse and practices are perceived as more central. This both limits and expands the ability of midwives to perform alternative constructions of birth care, as 'those symbols marked as central to society draw direct upon those powers amplified by the society's economy, institutions, and so on. Those marked as marginal are denied those powers but they also acquire access to those potencies suppressed by society' (Hariman 1999: 22).

As midwives attempt to move into the mainstream, they might acquire the powers of society while losing the power of the marginal. For example, as the midwives seek access through licensing, they must invoke the discourse of the dominant paradigm by reifying outcomes over more transcendental approaches to quality. Indeed, Turner (2002) found that when one group of midwives sought to discipline one of its members, the arguments used were grounded in conventional rather than alternative beliefs about quality. For example, when a midwife took a phone call during a birth, the others defined it as 'breaking the sterile field' rather than 'not being with the woman'. This was, however, the only argument that would generate a sanction by the licensing board. To live in both paradigms is problematic, but the response of the midwives to the technology paradox in the current study suggests an alternative.

Invoking multiple responses to a paradox might explode our meanings around specific concepts such as technology, midwifery and health care, thereby allowing alternative health care providers to operate in conventional settings while still embracing their beliefs in holism, inter-relationships and subjectivity. In this study, the midwives both narrow and broaden the meaning of technology. First, they narrow it to only specific situations. Second, they broaden it to allow them to participate in the use of technology more fully than do conventional birth care providers. Thus, midwives can still be the keepers of alternative birth ideologies yet participate in more conventional practices should the situation require. Should they be successful in redefining the meaning of technology, this could provide them with an entrée into conventional medical settings while retaining their own system of beliefs. However, because midwives will be defining these systems of meaning in conjunction with clients and conventional health care providers, future researchers should also examine the narratives of these stakeholders. The inclusion of dominant voices would provide a more fully developed understanding of the relationship of paradox, relations of power and what Foucault (1980) characterised as regimes of truth.

This chapter highlights that health care, health and the role of the provider are socially constructed and grounded in sometimes divergent beliefs that influence the intersection of CAM and conventional medicine. The reliance of conventional medicine on reductionism and objectivity appropriately sustain the need to find and fix a single meaning for health, health care and health care provider. Alternative birth care providers using CAM who attempt to move into conventional settings must find a way to negotiate the paradoxes that emerge when these fixed terms intersect with their own beliefs in plurality, holism and subjectivity. Specifically, in order to effectively mainstream alternative birthing care, we must also find ways to mainstream the possibility of multiple meanings for *health*, *health care* and *health care provider*.

Note

1 I have cited the statute verbatim to avoid identifying the state in which this centre operated and thereby protecting the privacy of study participants.

References

Barbato Gaydos, H. L. (2001) Complementary and alternative therapies in nursing education: trends and issues. *Online Journal of Issues in Nursing* 6(2): 5.

Berger, P. (1969) *A Rumor of Angels: Modern Society and the Rediscovery of the Supernatural*. Garden City, NY: Doubleday.

Chesebro, J. W. (1984) The symbolic construction of social realities: a case study in the rhetorical criticism of paradox. *Communication Quarterly* 32(2): 164–71.

Clair, R. P. (1996) The political nature of the colloquialism, 'a real job': implications for organisational socialisation. *Communication Monographs* 63(3): 249–67.

Clair, R. P., McGoun, M. J. and Spirek, M. M. (1993) Sexual harassment responses of working women: an assessment of current communication typologies and perceived effectiveness of the response. In Kreps, G. (ed.) *Sexual Harassment: Communication Implications*. Cresskill, NJ: Hampton, pp. 200–24.

Colton, D. (2000) Quality improvement in health care: conceptual and historical foundations. *Evaluation and the Health Professions* 23(1): 7–42.

Conquergood, D. (1991) Rethinking ethnography: towards a critical cultural politics. *Communication Monographs* 58(2): 179–94.

Conroy, R. M., Siriwardena, R., Smyth, O. and Fernandes, P. (2000) The relation of health anxiety and attitudes to doctors and medicine to use of alternative and complementary treatments in general practice patients. *Psychology, Health and Medicine,* 5(2): 203–13.

Coulter, I. (2004) Integration and paradigm clash: the practical difficulties of integrative medicine. In Tovey, P., Easthope, G. and Adams, J. (eds) *The Mainstreaming of Complementary and Alternative Medicine: Studies in Social Context*. London: Routledge, pp. 103–22.

Davis-Floyd, R. E. (1990) The role of obstetrical rituals in the resolution of cultural anomaly. *Social Science & Medicine* 31(2): 175–89.

de Beauvoir, S. (1961) *The Second Sex*, trans. H. M. Parshley. New York: Bantam.

Denzin, N. K. (2001) *Interpretive Interactionism*, 2nd edn. Thousand Oaks, CA: Sage.

Derrida, J. (1982) *Margins of Philosophy*. Chicago, IL: University of Chicago Press.

Donabedian, A. (1980) *The Definition of Quality and Approaches to Its Assessment*. Ann Arbor, MI: Health Administration Press.

Ehrenreich, B. and English, D. (1973) *Witches, Midwives, and Nurses: A History of Women Healers*. New York: Feminist Press.

Foucault, M. (1973) *The Birth of the Clinic: Archaeology of Medical Perception*, trans. A. M. S. Smith. New York: Vintage.

Foucault, M. (1980) *Power/Knowledge*, trans. C. Gordon. New York: Pantheon.

Foucault, M. (1990) *The History of Sexuality: An Introduction*, Vol. 1 trans. R. Hurley. New York: Vintage Books.

Fox, M. (1995) *The Reinvention of Work*. San Francisco, CA: HarperCollins.

Frohock, F. M. (2002) Moving lines and variable criteria: differences/connections between allopathic and alternative medicine. *Annals of the American Academy of Political and Social Science* 583(1): 214–32.

Gélis, J. (1991) *History of Childbirth*. Boston, MA: Northeastern University Press.

Grosz, E. (1994) *Volatile Bodies*. Indianapolis, IN: Indiana University Press.

Hariman, R. (1999) Radical sociality and Christian detachment in Erasmus' Praise of Folly. *World Order* 31: 9–23.

Jonas, W. B. (2002) Policy, the public, and priorities in alternative medicine research. *Annals of the American Academy of Political and Social Science* 583(1): 29–43.

Kligler, B. (1996) Challenges for the future: report on the first national conference on medical and nursing education in complementary therapies. *Journal of Alternative and Complementary Medicine* 2(4): 539–46.

Lohr, K. N. (1990) *Medicare: A Strategy for Quality Assurance*, Vol. 1. Washington, DC: Institute of Medicine, National Academy Press.

Lyotard, J. (1991) *The Postmodern Condition: A Report on Knowledge*. Minneapolis, MN: University of Minnesota Press.

Mitford, J. (1992) *The American Way of Birth*. New York: Penguin.

Moyad, M. A. (2001) The prevalence and effectiveness of complementary and alternative medicine: what has been learned and what it may be telling us about our patients, ourselves, and conventional medical treatment. *Seminars in Urologic Oncology* 19(4): 257–69.

Pollock, D. (1999) *Telling Bodies: Performing Birth*. New York: Columbia University Press.

Pursell, C. W., Jr (1980) History of technology. In Durbin, P. T. (ed.) *A Guide to the Culture of Science, Technology, and Medicine*. New York: Macmillan, pp. 70–120.

Putnam, L. L. (1983) Lady you're trapped: breaking out of conflict cycles. In Pilotta, J. J. (ed.) *Women in Organisations: Barriers and Breakthroughs*. Prospect Heights, IL: Waveland.

Reed, C. F., Pettigrew, A. C. and King, M. O. (2000) Alternative and complementary therapies in nursing curricula. *Journal of Nursing Education* 39(3): 133–9.

Sandelowski, M. (2002) Reembodying qualitative inquiry. *Qualitative Health Research* 12(1): 104–15.

Schreiber, L. (2005) The importance of precision in language: communication research and (so-called) alternative medicine. *Health Communication* 17(2): 173–90.

Scott, J. C. (1990) *Domination and the Arts of Resistance: Hidden Transcripts*. New Haven, CT: Yale University Press.

Smith, A. (1937) *The Wealth of Nations*. New York: Modem Library/Random House.

Stichler, J. F. and Weiss, M. E. (2001) Through the eye of the beholder: multiple perspectives on quality in women's health care. *Journal of Nursing Care Quality* 15(3): 59–74.

Thackray, A. (1980) History of science. in Durbin, P. T. (ed.) *A Guide to the Culture of Science, Technology, and Medicine*. New York: Macmillan, pp. 473–95.

Turner, P. K. (2002) Is childbirth with midwives natural? The gaze of the feminine and the pull of the masculine. *Qualitative Inquiry* 8(5): 652–69.

Varney, H. (1987) *Nurse-midwifery*, 2nd edn. Boston, MA: Blackwell Scientific.

Wendt, R. (1998) The sound of one hand clapping: counterintuitive lessons extracted from paradoxes and double binds in participative organizations. *Management Communication Quarterly* 11(3): 323–71.

Wertz, R. W. and Wertz, D. C. (1977) *Lying-in: A History of Childbirth in America*. New Haven, CT: Yale University Press.

White House Commission on Complementary and Alternative Medicine Policy (2002, March) Final Report (NIH Publication 03–5411). Washington, DC: Government Printing Office.

Wood, J. T. and Conrad, C. (1983) Paradox in the experiences of professional women. *Western Journal of Speech Communication* 47(4): 305–22.

Chapter 3

'Snake oil peddling': CAM and the occupational status of doctors and nurses

Peter Morrall

Introduction

On 25 October 2006 one of the headline stories run by the BBC news services was that leading scientific institutions in Britain had raised their concern that changes to the regulation of homeopathic medicines were putting patients at risk. At the same time the pro-science pressure group Sense About Science (SAS) reported that 600 medical practitioners and scientists, some of whom are leaders in their field, had signed a petition against allowing promoters of homeopathy to make medical claims about its efficacy (SAS 2006). SAS proclaims that evidence-based medicine is paramount to public health, and that there is no evidence that homeopathy contributes to public health (SAS 2006).

At around the same time as the SAS report, alterations to the rules governing what information can be provided to consumers of homeopathy had been made by Medicines and Healthcare products Regulatory Agency (MHRA). The chairperson of SAS, Lord Dick Taverne, commented:

> As many of the medical specialists contacting us have pointed out, evidence-based medicine has been a major public gain of the 20th Century. This is the first time, since the thalidomide tragedy and the 1968 Medicines Act, that the regulation of medicines has moved away from the science rather than towards it.
>
> (Taverne 2006)

The scientific organisations raising objections to these changes by the MHRA included: the Medical Research Council, the Royal College of Pathologists, the BioSciences Federation, the Physiological Society, the British Pharmacological Society, the Society for Applied Microbiology, the Royal Society and the Academy of Medical Sciences. In addition, hundreds of doctors and scientists have signed a statement opposing the rules allowing homeopathic medicines to make medical claims.

Nursing also claims to be an 'evidence-based' occupation (French 1999). But there was no equivalent outburst of concern from its formal organisations or leaders. Indeed, when it comes to complementary and alternative medicine (CAM), nursing has supported their promotion (both the scientifically legitimate varieties *and* treatments and practices that as yet remain unsubstantiated) to the degree that it seriously undermines its aspiration to become a full-fledged profession.

On 26 October 2006 the British press reported the comments of Sir John Oldham, Head of the Improvement Foundation which provides advice about National Health Service (NHS) policies, and a general practitioner:

> Doctors and nurses who fail to wash their hands although they know it reduces hospital infections are as bad as drunk drivers. . . . Sir John Oldham . . . warned that one in five hospital staff failed to wash their hands, despite evidence that doing so cuts the incidence of hospital acquired infections such as MRSA [methicillin-resistant staphylococcus aureus], which cost the NHS £1bn a year. Figures for 2004 show MRSA killed 1,168 patients in England and Wales.
>
> (Unattributed 2006)

Given that there is a wave of opinion, supported by some of the most senior judges and the Law Commission for drink driving to be included with a revised classification of illegal killing within English law (Morrall 2006) the accusation by Oldham is tantamount to accusing hospital staff of being guilty of homicide. Moreover, although under the rules of 'clinical governance' every health practitioner has the duty to act responsibly, it is nurses rather than doctors who have the primary responsibility for clinical cleanliness and infection control. Furthermore, if a doctor indulges in unhygienic practices and nurses believe they cannot challenge directly the medical miscreant, then this exemplifies the *sub*-professional status of nursing. Indeed, nurses engaging in unsubstantiated CAM can do nothing but threaten their present esteem.

In this chapter I first review what the scientific sceptics have to say about the credibility of CAM. Second, I review the credibility of scientific medicine to ascertain whether or not it has the epistemological and ethical authority to criticise CAM. Third, the respective stances taken by the profession of medicine and the discipline of nursing with regard to CAM are considered, and how their different positions affect their respective occupational status. I conclude that involvement with CAM is detrimental to the occupational standing of medicine *and* nursing. However, nurses are much more vulnerable to a reduction of prestige than medical practitioners because they are less cautious in their collusion with CAM. Moreover, I make the radical suggestion that nurses should concentrate on achieving success in basic care rather than extending their sphere of work to include CAM practice and treatment.

Sceptics

CAM, whether construed within the context of global capitalist expansionism or postmodern globalised consumer culture, have become fashionable and lucrative commodities (Tovey et al. 2004).

In the USA about one-third of the population visit CAM providers and in Germany CAM are used by 65 per cent of the population (Hirsch 2002). Studies in other countries have revealed similar prevalence rates (Adams et al. 2003; Barnes et al. 2004). Moreover, a multi-billion-pound international industry supports the production of CAM (Collyer 2004). For example, China MediTech, a traditional botanical drugs firm (which is developing ingredients to assist in the treatment of cancer and bowel disorders in the West as well as having an extensive health-supplements business in China) has 1,750 employees and was expected to be valued at at least £130 million in 2006 (Wray 2006).

Charles Windsor, Prince of Wales is in no doubt that CAM can make a substantial contribution to the delivery of health care in Britain. Windsor advocates what has become known as 'integrative medicine' – that is, the marriage of scientific medicine with CAM and he commissioned a report to investigate how CAM could be used within the NHS. The report, led by the economist Christopher Smallwood and aided by the research consultancy FreshMinds, was launched in 2005 (Smallwood 2005). Specifically, the research examined the prospective role of the 'big five' CAM modalities (osteopathy and chiropractic, acupuncture, homeopathy, and herbalism) in the NHS.

So, CAM is popular, and receives zealous support from the (potential) future King of England. But is CAM credible? To begin with the assimilation of CAM into mainstream health care is not merely a matter of convincing policy-makers and practitioners to do so. Placing CAM alongside scientific medicine and describing such an arrangement as integrative medicine cannot disguise fundamental contradictions between the two approaches. The philosophy and exercise of integrative medicine is radically different from that of scientific medicine (Coulter 2004). The former focuses on health and holism; the latter, on diagnosis and disease. Moreover, CAM is frequently underscored by an alternative not complementary epistemology to that of scientific medicine. In the main, scientific medicine uses empirical evidence (drawn from laboratory experiments and controlled randomised trials). Personal acclamation and Royal assertion is drawn on to back CAM:

As Patron of a number of health charities, The Prince of Wales has seen at first hand what a difference integrated healthcare has made for many people suffering from ill health.

(Windsor 2005)

Hirsch (2002) suggests that one way to regard the disparity between CAM and scientific medicine is to regard CAM as any therapy that has not been scientifically tested. By 'scientifically tested' Hirsch recommends the standard of 'rigorous evidence of safety and efficacy' set by USA Food and Drug Administration (FDA) before approval is given for any drug to be prescribed by medical practitioners. This is, of course, a teleological and self-serving position (Hirsch is, after all, a Professor of Medicine at University of Washington, USA). However, it does draw attention to how the issue of credibility is concerned with scientific verification (or the lack of it). Moreover, it is the inherent scepticism of science that marks the division between the 'belief' in CAM and the 'proof' of scientific medicine.

In order to explore this argument further we need to clarify: what is scepticism? First, the sceptic does not take anything at face value. Any and all propositions, no matter who submits them, are scrutinised. That is, the sceptic argues that nobody should be immune from such examination, whether he/she is Pope, Prime Minister, President, physicist, psychologist, pharmacist, homeopath, herbalist, or holist. Second, as Wendy Grossman (2006), editor of *The Skeptic* magazine, points out, to be sceptical is not to be negative but to search for the (scientific) evidence for any claim on truth, whether this is about creationism, intelligent-design, genetic function, superstring theory, M-theory, or colonic lavage. The work of Richard Dawkins (ultra-rationalist biologist and anti-religion crusader), Stephen Hawking (pre-eminent theoretical physicist and accomplished writer of popular science), as well as Sarah (fully qualified life coach and chartered accountant runs courses in total relaxation and meditation), and Barry (Whole Being Healing/Healer therapist) should all be evaluated critically.

CAM encompasses an amorphous and expanding collection of ailments, therapies and qualifications (Adams and Tovey 2004). Although tighter regulation of CAM has occurred or is in the offing in many Western countries, it remains relatively easy to declare oneself a 'healer' and distribute capriciously ointments for the mind and body, and courses that provide certificates to mete out CAM are proliferating.

Furthermore, what exactly is being referred to under the heading of CAM is not just an issue of the breadth of treatments and credentials. There is the problem of conflating tribal remedies and rituals of the witch-doctor or Shaman, and medieval religiosity and superstition with that of Eastern and Western traditional and modern healing practices (that is 'old-age' and 'new-age' philosophies, spiritualities, pills and potions). As commentators have suggested, in many cases the overriding commonality between many

CAMs is often no more than their mutual exclusion from mainstream health care (Adams and Tovey 2004).

What Windsor is advocating is the intertwining of two distinctive and incomparable epistemologies: (a) the reasoning from ancient civilisations of Mesopotamia, Egypt, Greece, Rome, and the European Renaissance, Enlightenment, and industrial epochs (Porter 2003); and (b) the convictions from a matrix of folklore, hocus-pocus, mysticism, and snake oil (Diamond 2001).

When investigative journalist John Diamond announced that he had contracted cancer he was inundated with advice to reject scientific medical treatment and use instead a 'miracle cure'. Rather than undergo chemotherapy it was suggested by thousands of people writing to him that he should try, for example, various herbs and nutritional supplements (Diamond 2001). Diamond became an arch sceptic, and his book *Snake Oil* (the foreword was written by Richard Dawkins) is a testament to that scepticism. What galled Diamond was the uncritical faith expressed by the letter writers in all things 'natural' and their detestation of what they regarded as 'synthetic' (that is, scientific) medicine.

The process of accommodating non-scientific health remedies within formal health care began in the latter part of the twentieth century when 'alternative' medicine mutated into 'complementary' medicine, later to be refashioned at the beginning of the twenty-first century as 'integrative' medicine (Konner 1993; Baer 2004). However, far from this representing a threat to the dominance and purity of scientific medicine the rebranding of 'alternative medicine' as 'complementary medicine' and again to 'integrative medicine' could be viewed as the successful colonisation of the challenger's territory rather than the triumphal infiltration of CAM into the domain of scientific medicine. Indeed, scientific medicine is progressing with taking possession of some CAMs. Those CAMs that have been scrutinised by scientific medicine, and have a demonstrable efficacy are incorporated by scientific medicine. Those that fail to demonstrate any efficacy are demonised, as is the case with homeopathy.

Of course assessing the merit of CAM using the rules of science is disingenuous if CAM purports an epistemological authority which is of a different nature to that of the laboratory experiment or randomised controlled double blind trial. However, the purveyors of CAM cannot have it both ways. It cannot be asserted logically in the defence of CAM that some are proven 'scientifically' to work, while those rejected by science are still of value due to the legitimacy of alternative models for understanding efficacy.

Edzard Ernst is probably the most prominent sceptic of CAM – a scepticism that could be considered bizarre given his position as Professor of Complementary Medicine at the Peninsula Medical School, Universities of Exeter and Plymouth. However, Ernst has a cogent view on CAM that emanates from his commitment to science. He is very critical of Windsor's campaign to have CAM integrated with scientific medicine (he originally participated in the investigation of CAM by the Smallwood team but later asked for his contribution to be withdrawn). He is therefore not in favour of the Prince of Wales' Foundation for Integrated Health which recruits general practitioners willing to offer a wide range of herbal and other CAM treatments to their patients. Ernst has signalled what he considers to be the dangers of the integrative approach recommended in the Smallwood Report (Ernst 2005).

> My professional life is dedicated to identifying what works in com-plementary medicine and, of course, I am in favour of using proven therapies. But probing beneath the surface of the UK initiatives for inte-grated medicine, one quickly finds problems.
>
> (Ernst 2005)

For example, Ernst cites the case of the natural remedy Devil's Claw, a shrub found in the Kalahari Desert, which has a similar analgesic effect to the synthetically produced paracetamol. The problem with using Devil's Claw, however, is that it has been over-harvested nearly to extinction, it is much more expensive than paracetamol, and it may have adverse interactions with other medication such as those given for cardio-vascular disease and as such Ernst argues that this 'natural' drug should not be supported.

Nevertheless, Ernst saves his raw scepticism for homeopathy. Shortly after the release of the Smallwood Report Ernst attacked the treatments already available through the NHS at five homeopathic hospitals:

> Homeopathic remedies don't work . . . Study after study has shown it is simply the purest form of placebo. You may as well take a glass of water than a homeopathic medicine . . . The incredibly dilute solutions used by homeopaths also make no sense . . . If it were true, we would have to tear up all our physics and chemistry textbooks.
>
> (Ernst in McKie 2005)

This is a view also expressed by Grossman in *The Skeptic* (2006). For Grossman there is a danger of returning to an era of superstition and pseudo-science in medicine. Moreover, she argues that just because something is popular doesn't make it credible.

Ernst insists that he is not against CAM *per se*, but wants to submit CAM to scientific scrutiny (Ernst 2005). Only the ones that have scientific validity can then be included in the lexicon of what he regards as legitimate medi-cines. For example, he accepts that some herbal remedies do work in a limited fashion. He admits that there is evidence that St John's Wort, acupuncture and hypnotherapy can work but suggests homeopathic treatments and chiropractic 'do no good' (Ernst in McKie 2005).

Medical practitioner, science writer and science campaigner for the *Guardian* newspaper, Ben Goldacre, has also been salaciously contemptuous about homeopathy over a period of years. Drawing attention to the weight of evidence disproving the efficacy of homeopathy, and agreeing with Ernst that its user-reported success is due to a placebo effect, Goldacre noted on the last day in 2005:

> My first new year's resolution is to write less about homeopaths, partly because teasing them is starting to bore me, and partly because we've won. Yes. Won. I'm talking about huge meta-analyses, summing together vast numbers of little trials, adding all the numbers up, and finding that overall, homeopathy is no better than placebo. That's not absence of evidence that it works. That's positive evidence that homeopathy does not work better than placebo.
>
> (Goldacre 2005)

Raymond Tallis, Professor of Geriatric Medicine, University of Manchester, is another arch sceptic with regard to CAM (Tallis 2004). He argues cogently that CAM does not avail itself to systematic critique in the same way that scientific medicine does. For Tallis, scientific medicine is in a constant state of dissatisfaction and transformation, seeking to find better understandings for disease and more pleasant treatments. On the other hand, far from discontent with its knowledge, CAM (due to its 'traditional' roots) is complacent and stagnant (Tallis 2004).

For Tallis the rising interest in CAM by both the public and health practitioners is having a corrupting effect on present medical achievements and on the possible triumph over disease (Tallis 2004). There is, argues Tallis, very little proof for the effectiveness of CAM other than the 'placebo effect', and the evidence that is provided is extremely dubious. He, like Diamond, regards CAM as analogous to snake oil:

> Of course there is much apparent evidence: anecdotes, patient testimony endorsements from satisfied customers – the kind of evidence used by the first huckster who sold his first bottle of *snake oil* off the back of his ox-cart and the first magician to turn his attention to the lucrative business of peddling cancer cures.
>
> (Tallis 2004: 128–9; emphasis added)

Tallis argues that CAM is no substitute for antibiotics, steroids, and modern pharmaceuticals which have proven their effectiveness in fighting cancer, alleviating heart dysfunction, and curing stomach ulcers. Moreover, Tallis observes how CAMs have become fashionable health products and practices primarily in affluent late modern societies, where consumers have the time and money to spend on what he views as 'whimsical' therapies (Tallis 2004). In the developing world people die or suffer in their tens of millions from diseases that could either be cured or assuaged by scientific medicine. Patients in the developing world, when knowledgeable about Western medicine, chose it above their traditional approaches (but of course only if they can afford to and have access to it). Support for traditional medicine in the West comes from misplaced sentimentality and obtuse cultural-relativism (Tallis 2004).

Tallis provides the example from his own experience of working as a medical practitioner in Nigeria. He recalls how affliction and death could have been prevented easily with the intervention of scientific medicine in Nigeria. However, ill-health was made worse and early death more likely (or even caused) by the administration of traditional remedies. He also highlights South African President Thabo Mbeki's original position on AIDS. In 2000, Mbeki refused to accept that AIDS was primarily a sexually transmitted disease caused by HIV infection which could be treated with Western drugs. Instead Mbeki argued that its prevalence had been exaggerated, denied knowing anyone with the disease, and insisted instead that AIDS was connected with impoverished lifestyles. With regard to traditional medicine, Mbeki's health minister Manto Tshabalala-Msimang went as far as to suggest that those with HIV should eat beetroot and garlic. However, in the face of public disquiet at home and internationally about his views and ex-president Nelson Mandela's open support for scientific medication, Mbeki stopped pronouncing on the subject. By the end of 2006 Manto Tshabalala-Msimang had been sidelined politically and the South African Government had abandoned its beetroot and garlic advice in favour of anti-retroviral medication (BBC News 2006).

Science

The medical profession has an inexorable link with science – science has been adopted by medicine for hundreds of years as 'ideological ammunition' (Morgan et al. 1985). Science gives medicine its perceived integrity, an integrity furthered by constant radical innovations in physics, chemistry, mathematics, computer technology, molecular and cell biology, genetics, and pharmacology. *Scientific* medicine has spread rapaciously and ubiquitously, furnishing the dual processes of medicalisation and professionalisation. But how credible is scientific medicine and science itself?

Tallis has an absolutist stance: you're either for or against scientific medicine (Tallis 2004). However, Tallis's rigid view has found criticism (Whitaker 2004). Whitaker argues that the evidence supporting scientific medicine is skewed considerably. Specifically, pharmaceutical corporations are the major financial backers of medical research through clinical trials. Whitaker argues that it is not surprising, therefore, that the treatments doctors prescribe are mainly pharmaceutical products – other commentators have outlined similar positions (e.g. Cohen 2007).

Whitaker also observes that although Tallis appreciates the limited role of medical science in the dramatic improvements to health and life expectancy within Britain from the nineteenth century onwards, he seems to ignore the potential for further improvements to medical science. That is, social, political and economic policies can again make radical differences to morbidity and mortality rates rather than medical knowledge. But effective medical care is still required to assuage disease and thwart death while waiting for those policies to be implemented. This is especially so in areas of the world where social, political and economic changes may be on their way but malaria, tuberculosis, HIV/AIDS have already arrived. Moreover, if and when such policies are fully in force there will still be an array of residual health issues (and new ones arising) that require medical attention.

There are certainly many ethical questions concerning the manipulation of medical practice. For example, the pharmaceutical companies manoeuvre medical practice through blatant inducements. These range from complimentary boiled sweets and ice cream at medical conferences, computer hardware and exotic holidays, glossy advertisements in medical journals, and the deployment of armies of 'reps' to push their companies' medicinal wares. More subtle manipulation is the paying for the research papers to be 'ghost-written' in a manner that hides negative effects of the particular pharmaceutical company's products or promotes its new products. Prestigious medical academics and practitioners are then asked to add their names to these papers to strengthen their chances of being accepted as authentic by the wider medical community (Fugh-Berman 2005).

Lisa Cosgrove and her collaborators (2006) investigated the financial links between the members of the panel responsible for revision in diagnostic criteria within the widely used American Psychiatric Association's diagnostic manual (the DSM-IV), and the pharmaceutical industry. What Cosgrove et al. discovered was that over half of the panel members had one or more such links. Pharmaceutical corporations had monetary arrangements with *all* members of the panels on 'Mood Disorders' and 'Schizophrenia and Other Psychotic Disorders'. Commenting on the research, bioethicist Mildred Cho, from Stanford University in California, makes the point that the pharmaceutical corporations have a vested interest in the adjudication of psychiatric categories as the existence of a disorder will usually mean there is a demand for their drug treatments (Cho in Aldhous 2006).

Beyond these commercial manipulations, the political misuse of scientific evidence has been highlighted by the British Parliamentary Select Committee on Science and Technology (SCST). Chairman Phil Willis (Willis 2006), reporting the findings of the report by the SCST 'Scientific Advice, Risk and Evidence Based Policy Making', criticised government Ministers for selling their policies to media and public on false pretences. Willis accepts that not every policy has to be bolstered by science, but he accused Ministers of presenting certain policies as having scientific substantiation when they do not. For Willis, the difference between 'conviction-based policies' and 'evidence-based policies' should be made crystal clear through the publication of the scientific data and advice whenever it is available (Willis 2006).

Along with unethical *modus operandi* of pharmaceutical companies, the standing of the underpinning epistemology of medical practice (that is, science) can be questioned. The philosopher Karl Popper (1959), the historian Thomas Kuhn (1962), and subsequently the sociologists of scientific knowledge, have highlighted the social processes involved in, and the fallibility of, scientific endeavour (Fuller 1997).

Karl Popper's thesis was that science is not united over how to go about collecting and testing 'facts'. For Popper science cannot establish permanent truths; rather than science proclaiming to 'prove' the existence of facts, Popper reinterpreted the mission of science as aiming to falsify correlations between variables (such as smoking and lung cancer, eating fatty foods and high blood cholesterol, or arnica and inflammation) (Popper 1959). Each test of falsification either weakens a suggested link between variables or implies that this link can be taken as valid, but only for as long as a subsequent test is not invented that then refutes the link (Popper 1959).

Kuhn (1962) argues that scientists operate within a 'paradigm' that is accepted as legitimate by the scientific community. During the period that Kuhn calls 'normal science' scientists merely address particular problems that are internally consistent with that paradigm. That is, only those problems that have an indubitable connection with the principles of the paradigm are researched. Conclusions from research can only be plausible when they are coterminous with those principles. Any evidence produced during 'normal science' that contradicts the precepts of the accepted paradigm is dispensed with through ridicule. Alternatively, they are contained through the production of theories that are in tune with the paradigm. However, periodically there is such a build-up of evidence repudiating the paradigm that it starts to disintegrate. According to Kuhn, the period of 'normal science' then ends and 'revolutionary science' begins. The revolutionary period is a time of epistemological turmoil due to competing claims over what can be considered authentic knowledge. Eventually, the turmoil ends and a modified paradigm or completely novel paradigm emerges.

It could be that the popularity of CAM (along with, for example, the 'dangerous' growth in religious fanaticism [Dawkins 2006]) signifies the commencement of revolutionary epistemological epoch. While it is unlikely that CAM will replace medical science, 'integrated medicine' might be a modifying force leading to a new 'normal science' (Cohen 2007).

Much more extreme than either Popper or Kuhn is the postmodernist critique of truth (Lash 1990). Postmodernist reasoning takes an ultra-relativist position. Whether it is CAM, scientific medicine, quantum mechanics, superstring/M-theory, Buddhism, Judaism, Christianity, Islamism, humanism, cognitive-behaviourism, holism, socialism, capitalism, rationalism, any 'truth' is considered as good as all others. Postmodern life is made up from a multitude of possible truths in a world where everything has been fashioned into a commodity. We may, as health consumers, combine the treatments from our general practitioner with advice from the health food shop-assistant, obtain statins from the consultant cardiologist or Jiang Ya Ping Pian from the Chinese herbalist, swallow a Viagra tablet or learn to flex our Tantric 'love muscle'.

However, a realist position about science, and one to which I subscribe, acknowledges that the methods of science have to be seen for what they are (inexact), as well as influenced by extraneous factors. But the acknowledgement of uncertainty in science is not the same as arguing that science is worthless. Moreover, viewing science as inexact, and therefore frequently misleading in its interpretation of the social and natural realms, should not lead automatically to the conclusion that these realms can be better elucidated by substitute epistemologies, or cannot ever be explained by science.

Simon Blackburn (Professor of Philosophy at Cambridge University) is not a scientific purist. However, he makes an incisive observation about reality:

> Prince Charles never flies a helicopter burning homeopathically diluted petrol, that is water with only a memory of benzene molecules, maintained by a schedule derived from reading tea leaves, and navigated by a crystal ball.
>
> (Blackburn 2006: 196)

For Blackburn we should respect the authority and goal of scientific truth while remaining sceptical about future developments. Finding what was once considered the truth no longer can be sustained does not negate the search for the real truth. His brand of realism leads him to conclude:

> . . . retain our hard-won confidences [from natural and social scientific endeavour], without closing our minds to any further illuminations that the future may bring . . . Above all, I hope, we have become confident in using our well-tried and tested vocabulary of explanation and assessment. We can take the postmodernist inverted commas off things that ought to matter to us: truth, reason, objectivity and confidence.
>
> (Blackburn 2006: 221)

Given the faults of science, what does the best science available indicate about CAM? The British Government's database for health research is the National Library for Health. A search through this database reveals that the scientific evidence for CAM can be placed in one of three categories:

(a) some are not supported by sufficient scientific evidence to warrant their use in the NHS (for example, aromatherapy for dementia – Thorgrimsen et al., 2003; acupuncture for schizophrenia – Rathbone and Xia 2005; cranberries for urinary tact infections – Jepson et al., 2004; Ginkgo Biloba for cognitive impairment and dementia – Birks and Grimley Evans 2002; homeopathy for anything – Shang et al. 2005);
(b) others are fuelling dangerous health care practices (herbal medicines for treating HIV infection and AIDS – Liu et al. 2005);
(c) a few are dangerous in their own right because of adulteration (for example, Chinese herbs – Ernst 2002). There are exceptions. In particular, scientific evidence exists to indicate St John's Wort *may* be effective for treating mild to moderate depression (Linde et al. 2005).

Status

Medicine is perceived by the public as the most trustworthy of professions (Morrall 2001; IPSOS MORI 2006). Nursing is not a profession, and public perception includes subordination to doctors, low academic standards, limited career opportunities and poor pay and conditions (Morrall 2001; Brodie et al. 2004). Both medicine and nursing purport to base their practice on (scientific) 'evidence'. While medicine has little quarrel with such a commitment, the commitment of nursing to science is ambiguous. At times nursing presents itself as an 'art' rather than (or as well as) a science (Clarke 1999), or attempts to amalgamate the two (Ramey and Bunkers 2006). Moreover, nursing research has tended to ally itself with 'soft science' (that is, qualitative design) rather than 'hard science' (that is, quantitative design) (Holloway and Wheeler 2002).

Crucially, in terms of occupational status, medicine is much more circumspect about threats to its scientific credibility than nursing. For example, spokespersons for the Royal College of General Practitioners and the British Medical Association (BMA) have publicly warned medical practitioners to be aware that evidence to support the use of some CAM is lacking (BBC News 2005). An in-house editorial in the prestigious medical journal *The Lancet* (Horton 2005) called for the banning of the use of homeopathy in the NHS, and this was reported widely in the press. The acronym 'TEETH', provided by medical practitioner Adam Fox, is an example of a common medical colloquialism indicative of medical scepticism about at least one CAM:

TEETH – Tried Everything Else, Try Homeopathy.

(Fox 2003)

Undoubtedly doctors are recommending CAM, and do lead specialist CAM health care units. For example, the Bristol Homeopathic Hospital employs two NHS consultants and seven clinical assistants (King 2005). For 150 years the Royal London Homeopathic Hospital has been the largest public sector hospital for integrated complementary and alternative medicine in Europe. Conventional medical training schools now include information about CAM in undergraduate curricula (House of Lords 2000).

Meanwhile, nurses are using CAM more and more, both under the direct control of the medical profession and as primary prescribers (either with or without medical sanction), in both primary care and hospitals (Peters et al. 2001; Snyder and Lindquist 2002). Nursing courses in CAM have been founded in countries such as the UK, Australia, and the USA (Melland and Clayburn 2000).

Nevertheless, while both nursing and the medical profession are increasingly incorporating CAM, nurses are more likely than doctors to indulge in those 'therapies' that fall outside scientific validation. Moreover, there is a major difference between the responses of the medical establishment to CAM compared with that of nursing.

In 2006, thirteen eminent medical scientists (six of whom are fellows of the Royal Society) sent an open letter to the Chief Executive of St George's Healthcare NHS Trust in London, detailing their concerns about CAM being used in the NHS (Times Online 2006). The letter, published in the press, refers to the 'unproven' or 'disproved' CAM infiltrating health care in Britain, and asking the Chief Executive to join them in representing their concerns to the Department of Health. Professor David Read, the Vice-president of the Royal Society, gave support to the concerns expressed in the letter (quoted in Boseley 2006).

Although it may have been a more obvious role for the British nurses' (and midwives') regulatory body organisation, the Nursing and Midwifery Council (NMC), the Royal College of Nursing (RCN) has taken the lead role in the attempt to provide coherent direction over the use of CAM (RCN 2006). However, advice about nurses using CAM is currently confused and unclear. The NMC's position is that it has no responsibility for CAM practitioners, nor the scope to provide specific advice training for nurses in CAM (NMC 2006). The RCN's position is to offer a framework to ensure that nurses follow their professional code of conduct when using CAM in their practice. The professional code of practice is the responsibility of the NMC (NMC 2002). The RCN's specific guidance is that it is the responsibility of the individual practitioner to judge whether she/he is suitably qualified and competent to prescribe CAM. If working independently, then the nurse must monitor her/his own performance. If working in the NHS, then she/he should discuss the use of CAM with colleagues, principally the relevant medical practitioner and pharmacist. The RCN, however, recognises that there is a lack of policy within the NHS to support the integration of CAM into health care, and a wide variation in education about the safe use of CAM (RCN 2006).

The General Medical Council (GMC), on the other hand, is much clearer in its guidance about CAM (GMC 2006). It states that medical practitioners can prescribe 'unlicensed' medicines but must: be satisfied first that that a 'licensed' medicine would not meet the patient's needs; be satisfied that there is a sufficient evidence base and/or experience of using the medicine to demonstrate its safety and efficacy; take responsibility for prescribing the unlicensed medicine and for overseeing the patient's care (GMC 2006).

The BMA (2006) goes further. General practitioners are obliged under their contracts with primary care organisations (PCOs) to refer patients for services available under the NHS, and referral to complementary therapists should not therefore be considered a contractual requirement (the exception is referral to one of the five NHS homeopathic hospitals). Many general practitioners, the BMA points out, may not feel able to advise a patient to consult a complementary therapist and will therefore not wish to make such a referral. The BMA warns that if the referred patient suffers any harm as a result of treatment given by the CAM practitioner, then the general practitioner could retain some liability. Moreover, if delegating to a CAM practitioner (who perhaps is employed by the general practitioner), then the BMA makes clear that the general practitioner remains responsible for the patient's care.

Conclusion

The use of CAM by the profession of medicine could damage its occupation status because it deviates from its scientific heritage. As this chapter illustrates, both individual medical practitioners and medical organisations have assumed a sceptical stance towards CAM in line with this scientific heritage. Furthermore, contemporary revolutionary scientific developments are offering the medical profession enhanced ideological ammunition, thereby assuring its professional credibility.

Nursing is not so sceptical about CAM because, despite its claim to uphold evidence-based practice, it has no such loyalty to science. Un-sceptical acceptance of CAM by nursing, I suggest, *will* damage its occupational status. It has been argued for decades that such primary functions of nursing as 'hygiene' are being lost (Watson 1981), and research indicates that a lack of hygiene persists when patients are known to carry deadly infectious disease (Jenner et al. 2006). Claire Rayner, social campaigner and former nurse, who contracted MRSA while undergoing surgery, compares how she was trained as a nurse with contemporary nursing practice:

We scrubbed everything. When a patient was discharged, the bed was scoured from top to bottom, including the mattress, to make it fit for the next patient. And we scrubbed ourselves too. We washed our hands 40 or more times a day. We changed our uniforms if the slightest smear of blood or other body fluid marked it. We never left the hospital in uniform, never wore makeup and had to manicure our fingernails every week, without polish of course, for which sister inspected us each morning. And we never had any cross-infection among our patients. And now? Nurses no longer scrub and clean patients' equipment and – dare I say it – themselves, as we used to. There are no longer scary sisters or all-powerful matrons with the power to insist on the rules of cleanliness for all, including ward maids and orderlies who did even more cleaning than we did. And now there is a great deal of cross-infection, some of it capable of killing patients.

(Rayner 2004)

Rather than nurses indulging in unsubstantiated CAM ('snake oil peddling'), I suggest that their occupational status would be improved if they peddled *nursing*.

References

Adams, J., Easthope, G., Sibbritt, D. and Young, A. (2003) The profile of women who consult alternative health practitioners in Australia. *Medical Journal of Australia* 179(6): 297–300.

Aldous, P. (2006) Do drug firm links sway psychiatry? *New Scientist* 2549, 29 April: 14.

Baer, H. A. (2004) *Toward an Integrative Medicine*. Blue Ridge Summit, PA: Rowman & Littlefield.

Barnes, P., Powell-Griner, E., McFann, K. and Nahin, R. L. (2004) Complementary and alternative medicine use among adults: United States, 2002. *Advance Data* 27(343): 1–19.

BBC News (2005) Public 'back alternative therapy', 25 January: http://news.bbc.co.uk/go/pr/fr/-/1/hi/health/4203479.stm

BBC News (2006) SA launches plan to combat Aids, 1 December: http://news.bbc.co.uk/1/hi/world/africa/6200308.stm

Birks, J. and Grimley Evans, J. (2002) Ginkgo Biloba for cognitive impairment and dementia. *The Cochrane Database of Systematic Reviews* Issue 4. Art. No.: CD003120. DOI: 10.1002/14651858.CD003120.

Blackburn, S. (2006) *Truth: A Guide for the Perplexed*. London: Penguin.

BMA (British Medical Association) (2006) Referrals to complementary therapists: http://www.bma.org/

Boseley, S. (2006) Doctors' letter sparks NHS alternative therapies row. *Guardian*, 24 May.

Brodie, D., Andrews, G., Andrews, J., Thomas, G., Wong, J. and Rixon, L. (2004) Perceptions of nursing: confirmation, change and the student experience. *International Journal of Nursing Studies* 41(7): 721–33.

Clarke, L. (1999) Nursing in search of a science: the rise and rise of the new nurse brutalism. *Mental Health Care* 2(8): 270–2.

Cohen, M. (2007) Evidence and CAM research: challenges and opportunities. In Adams, J. (ed.) *Researching Complementary and Alternative Medicine*. London: Roultedge.

Collyer, F. (2004) The corporatisation and commercialisation of CAM. In Tovey, P., Easthope, G. and Adams, J. (eds) *The Mainstreaming of Complementary and Alternative Medicine: Studies in Social Context*. London: Routledge, pp. 81–99.

Cosgrove, L., Krimsky, S., Vijayaraghavana, M. and Schneidera, L. (2006) Financial ties between DSM-IV panel members and the pharmaceutical industry. *Psychotherapy and Psychosomatics* 75(3): 154–60.

Coulter, I. (2004) Integration and paradigm clash: the practical difficulties of integrative medicine. In Tovey, P., Easthope, G. and Adams, J. (eds) *The Mainstreaming of Complementary and Alternative Medicine: Studies in Social Context*. London: Routledge, pp. 103–22.

Dawkins, R. (2006) *The God Delusion*. London: Bantam.

Diamond, J. (2001) *Snake Oil and Other Preoccupations*, foreword Richard Dawkins; ed. Dominic Lawson. London: Vintage.

Ernst, E. (2002) Adulteration of Chinese herbal medicines with synthetic drugs: a systematic review. *Journal of Internal Medicine* 252: 107–13.

Ernst, E. (2005) Integral risk. *Guardian*, 16 August.

Fox, A. (2003) Doctor slang is a dying art. BBC News, 18 August: http://news.bbc.co.uk/go/pr/fr/-/1/hi/health/3159813.stm

French, P. (1999) The development of evidence-base nursing. *Journal of Advanced Nursing* 29(1): 72–8.

Fugh-Berman, A. (2005) Not in my name: how I was asked to 'author' a ghost-written research paper. *Guardian*, 21 April.

Fuller, S. (1997) *Science*. Buckingham: Open University Press.

Goldacre, B. (2005) Homeopathy: someone should tell the government that there's nothing in it. *Guardian*, 31 December.

Grossman, W. (2006) Comments on alternative medicine: www.skeptic.org.uk/medicine.html

Hirsch, I. B. (2002) Unproven therapies. *Clinical Diabetes* 20: 1–3.

Holloway, I. and Wheeler, S. (2002) *Qualitative Research in Nursing*. Oxford: Blackwell.

Horton, R. (2005) (editorial) The end of homeopathy. *The Lancet* 336, 27 August–2 September: 690.

House of Lords (2000) *Science and Technology – Sixth Report*. London: HMSO.

IPSOS MORI (2006) Public trust in doctors is still high: www.ipsos-mori.com/polls/2006/rcp.shtml

Jenner, E., Fletcher, B., Watson, P., Jones, F., Miller, L. and Scott, G. (2006) Discrepancy between self-reported and observed hand hygiene behaviour in healthcare professionals. *Journal of Hospital Infection* 63(4), August: 418–22.

Jepson, R. G., Mihaljevic, L. and Craig, J. (2004) Cranberries for preventing urinary tract infections. *The Cochrane Database of Systematic Reviews* Issue 2. Art. No.: CD001321. DOI: 10.1002/14651858.CD001321.

King, C. (2005) Bristol Homeopathic Hospital Outpatient Department Co-ordinator: Personal communication by email.

Konner, M. (1993) *The Tangled Wing: Biological Constraints on the Human Spirit.* Harmondsworth: Penguin Sciences.

Kuhn, T. (1962) *The Structure of Scientific Revolutions.* Chicago, IL: University of Chicago Press.

Lash S. (1990) *The Sociology of Postmodernism.* London: Routledge.

Linde, K., Mulrow, C. D., Berner, M. and Egger, M. (2005) St John's Wort for depression. *The Cochrane Database of Systematic Reviews* Issue 3. Art. No.: CD000448. DOI: 10.1002/14651858.CD000448.

Liu, J. P., Manheimer, E. and Yang, M. (2005) Herbal medicines for treating HIV infection and AIDS. *The Cochrane Database of Systematic Reviews* Issue 3. Art. No.: CD003937. DOI: 10.1002/14651858.CD003937.

McKie, R. (2005) Professor savages homeopathy. *Observer*, 18 December.

Melland, H. I. and Clayburn, T. L. (2000) Complementary therapies: introduction into a nursing curriculum. *Nurse Educator* 25(5): 247–50.

Morgan, M., Calnan, M. and Manning, N. (1985) *Sociological Approaches to Health and Medicine.* London: Croom Helm.

Morrall, P. (2001) *Sociology and Nursing.* London: Routledge.

Morrall, P. (2006) *Murder and Society.* Chichester: Wiley.

National Library for Health (2006) www.library.nhs.uk/default.aspx

NMC (Nursing and Midwifery Council) (2002) *Code of Professional Conduct.* London: NMC.

NMC (Nursing and Midwifery Council) (2006) Complementary therapies position statement – January 1999 (Updated 2002): http://www.nmc-uk.org/

Peters, D., Chaitow, L., Morrison, S. and Harris, G. (2001) *Integrating Complementary Therapies in Primary Care: A Practical Guide for Health Professionals.* Edinburgh: Churhill Livingstone.

Popper, K. (1959) *The Logic of Scientific Discovery.* New York: Harper and Row.

Porter, R. (2003) *Blood and Guts: A Short History of Medicine.* London: Penguin.

Ramey, S. and Bunkers, S. (2006) Teaching the abyss: living the art-science of nursing. *Nursing Science Quarterly* 19(4): 311–15.

Rathbone, J. and Xia, J. (2005) Acupuncture for schizophrenia. *The Cochrane Database of Systematic Reviews* Issue 4. Art. No.: CD005475. DOI: 10.1002/14651858.CD005475.

Rayner, C. (2004) Hospitals need a good scrub: modern-day nurses should have old-style mentors to teach them the basics of hygiene. *Guardian*, 11 October.

RCN (Royal College of Nursing) (2006) *Complementary Therapies in Nursing, Midwifery and Health Visiting Practice: RCN Guidance on Integrating Complementary Therapies into Clinical Care.* London: RCN.

SAS (Sense About Science) (2006) Statement on Evidence-based Medicine and The Medicines for Human Use (National Rules for Homeopathic Products) Regulations 2006: www.senseaboutscience.org.uk/

Shang, A. S., Huwiler-Müntener, K., Nartey, L., Jüni, P., Dörig, S., Sterne, J. A. C., Pewsner, D. and Egger, M. (2005) Are the clinical effects of homeopathy placebo effects? Comparative study of placebo-controlled trials of homeopathy and allopathy. *The Lancet* 336, 27 August–2 September: 726–32.

Smallwood, C. (2005) *The Role of Complementary and Alternative Therapy in the NHS*. London: FreshMinds Consultancy.

Snyder, M. and Lindquist, R. (eds) (2002) *Complementary/Alternative Therapies in Nursing*. New York: Springer

Stein, L. (1967) The doctor-nurse game. *Archives of General Psychiatry* 16: 699–703.

Tallis, R. (2004) *Hippocratic Oaths: Medicine and Its Discontents*. London: Atlantic.

Taverne, D. (2006) Quoted in BBC News: Scientists attack homeopathy move, 25 October: http://news.bbc.co.uk/1/hi/health/6085242.stm

Thorgrimsen, L., Spector, A., Wiles, A. and Orrell, M. (2003) Aroma therapy for dementia. *The Cochrane Database of Systematic Reviews* Issue 3. Art. No.: CD003150. DOI: 10.1002/14651858.CD003150.

Times Online (2006) Doctors' campaign against alternative therapies, 23 May: http://www.timesonline.co.uk/

Tovey, P., Easthope, G. and Adams, J. (eds) (2004) *The Mainstreaming of Complementary and Alternative Medicine: Studies in Social Context*. London: Routledge.

Unattributed (2006) Flounting of NHS hygiene 'as bad as drink driving'. *Guardian*.

Watson, J. (1981) The lost art of nursing. *Nursing Forum* 20(3): 244–9.

Whitaker, P. (2004) Patience, patients. *Guardian*, 30 October.

Willis, P. (2006) Publication of Report by the Selection Committee on Science and Technology, *Scientific Advice, Risk and Evidence Based Policy Making*. No. 63 of Session 2005–06 8 November October: www.parliament.uk/parliamentary_committees/science_and_technology_committee/scitech081106.cfm

Windsor, C., Prince of Wales (2005) Christopher Smallwood's Report on Integrated Health, 6 October: www.princeofwales.gov.uk/news/2005/10.oct/smallwood.php

Wray, R. (2006) First Chinese medicine firm floats in London to fund research. *Guardian*, 10 April.

Part II

Intra-professional issues

Chapter 4

The authentication of CAM in nursing

An examination of historic referencing in selected nursing journals

Philip Tovey and Jon Adams

Introduction

Membership figures for the UK Royal College of Nursing (RCN) Complementary Therapies Forum illustrate the surge of interest in complementary and alternative medicine (CAM) within the profession: 1,600 in 1997; rising to 11,400 in 2000 (House of Lords 2000) and the activities of similar representative bodies in other developed countries have confirmed this trend on the international stage (Fox-Young 1998; RCNA 1997). This is occurring at an interesting time in the development of nursing more broadly, given the ongoing attention to an enhanced nursing role, and continuing debate about the profession's most appropriate form and content (Barton 1999). It is a debate in which the essence of nursing is contested and recourse to history frequently undertaken in an attempt to legitimise specific conceptions of nursing (Hall and Allan 1994; Hisama 1996; Rinker 2000; Salmore 1998; Snyder and Lindquist 2001; Watson 1998; Wilson 2000).

Crucially, just as the nature of nursing as a whole is a matter of debate, so too is the role of CAM within it. The unprecedented expansion of interest should not be conflated with consensus. There is a clear line of thinking which is critical of its integration within nursing (Giuffe 1997), and this is coupled with continuing scepticism within medicine (Bartholomew and Likely 1998; Dew 2000; Federspil and Vettor 2000; Levin 1996). Thus, as a consequence, one important aspect of the current CAM nursing context is the pressure to advocate, legitimise or at least defend integration. And, despite the persistent talk of mainstreaming, practical examples of utilisation develop in a largely *ad hoc* manner. There is nothing pre-determined about an ever-increasing integration and expansion of available modalities.

This chapter has two closely related aims. First, to argue for a preliminary position that *nostalgia referencing and nostophobic referencing* (defined below) constitute one set of useful conceptual tools necessary to help develop a sociology of CAM in relation to nursing. We argue that *nostalgic and nostophobic referencing* are identifiable rhetorical strategies being used by authors advocating CAM/nursing integration. Authors are presenting a view of the history of nursing that is partial (selective), at times romanticised and open to debate. These presentations are composed in such a way as to identify a seamless connection between, on the one hand, what nursing has been, is, should be (and at times has been prevented from being); and, on the other, the character of CAM. We suggest that the utilisation of such strategies can be understood in terms of the need that CAM nursing has to authenticate and legitimise its (sub-world) specific view of nursing against a background of intra- and inter-professional contestation over the shape and direction of nursing. Our second aim is to suggest that these concepts have the potential for ongoing utility in future empirical research within the emerging sociology of CAM and nursing. We draw on evidence from an exploratory analysis of texts published from within the nursing community to support our case.

Conceptual background

Nostalgia and nostophobia

Nostalgia, both as a loose description and as a more tightly defined concept, has appeared in a range of sociological literature. It has been used in analyses of cultural shifts, notably the popularisation of heritage (Gabriel 1993), and not unconnectedly in analyses of social action within organisations – especially the workplace (Strangleman 1999). For instance, it has been argued that during periods of organisational change, the past is called upon as a representation of something altogether better, a point of comparison with an uncertain or unsatisfactory present (Gabriel 1993). More recently, discussion of nostalgia has appeared in a range of contexts including ecology (Mukta and Hardiman 2000) and immigrant experience (Lomsky-Feder and Rapoport 2000). Crucially, it is acknowledged that the use of nostalgia is neither neutral nor benign for those so engaged (Woolley 1999). However, to date its use in the context of health and health care has been almost non-existent (Abel 1986; Lupton 2000).

The concept of nostophobia (Davis 1979) is less frequently used. It is a potentially useful flip side to nostalgia: an assessment of the past as essentially negative, and of the future as an opportunity to rectify its limitations. Thus, following earlier writers, we see the concept as 'useful in analysing the way organisational members reverse the positive/negative temporal division and see the past as an era to be escaped from, and the new, more positive one, actively embraced' (Strangleman 1999: 727–8). The incorporation of both nostophobic and nostalgic representations of the past enables our analysis to chart the *flexible* use of historical referencing – a particular feature of discourse more generally which has been shown to add strength to the performance of an account (Gilbert and Mulkay 1984; Kerr et al. 1997).

One particularly interesting treatment of *nostalgia* is presented by Turner (1987). Here the author discusses both the role of nostalgia in Western civilisation as a whole and its place in modern social theory. Turner argues for a four-fold conceptualisation of a nostalgic paradigm. This (nostalgic) discourse is characterised by: a sense of historical decline with an associated movement away from a 'golden age of homefulness' (p. 150); the loss of 'personal wholeness and moral certainty' (p. 150); a sense of the individual operating within a rationalised structure, one devoid of meaningful and genuine social relationships; and, 'the loss of simplicity, personal authenticity and emotional spontaneity' (p. 150). While the author's concern is with macro-level developments, as will become clear, public presentations of CAM nurses draw heavily on strikingly similar rhetorics.

Social worlds and rhetorics

While it is important to develop conceptual tools specific enough to reflect the complexity of nursing culture, structure and history, this does not demand the wholesale rejection of existing CAM sociology. Indeed, our analysis draws on aspects of a theoretical framework recently introduced for the study of the medical appropriation of CAM – social worlds theory (SWT) (Tovey and Adams 2001). SWT has been detailed at length previously and here we limit discussion to the most directly relevant dimensions of the framework.

The theory is based on a conceptualisation of society as being made up of multiple social worlds, each of which is essentially inter-connected. Of importance here is the theoretical assertion of the inevitability of the fragmentation of these worlds into sub-worlds, and that such sub-worlds will be actively engaged in processes that are geared towards establishing worth and validity.

Crucial to such attempts to gain validity and worth are the rhetorics of worlds and their sub-worlds. Indeed, worlds are themselves constituted and reconstituted by rhetorical practices and have been conceptualised as 'universes of discourse' by earlier theorists (Shibutani 1955). Examining the different worlds of health care draws attention to 'representational practices' (Opie 1997) (whether in the public arena or more informal settings) and also highlights the inherently political dimension to these practices as groups attempt to gain epistemic authority, raise their market profile and attract or maintain financial resources for their world.

CAM nursing can appropriately be seen in these terms and rhetorics employed in such public presentations as the journal texts analysed here can be seen as constituting attempts by those within the sub-world of CAM nursing to accrue validity and authentication for their 'new found' practices and technologies. SWT provides concepts through which these processes can be considered. One such concept is *authentication* (Strauss

1982). This concept refers to the processes by which sub-groups justify non-traditional practices to others in their professional community. It is about establishing legitimacy and ultimately 'asking for a deserved place in the firmament of the larger social world' (Strauss 1982: 175). Attempts at *authentication* are pivotal to the research presented in this chapter.

A key strength of a social worlds perspective is its attention to processual change and, furthermore, its insistence that an understanding of any contemporary world must include an examination of the fluidity and transfiguration of that world (and others in the same arena) over a designated historical period (Clarke 1990; 1991). Indeed, Strauss – often perceived as the main promoter of SWT – highlights the importance of analysing the 'full historical development' of social worlds (Strauss 1978: 202) and reminds us that the very history of a world is itself constituted and reconstituted through the *claims-making activities* of world members (Strauss 1982).

While social world theorists' interest in historical analysis underscores our focus upon nostalgic and nostophobic referencing, previous work has not examined the role of historical referencing strictly in terms of world members' representational practices. In this sense, the present work develops a fresh approach to historical analysis from within a social world perspective. It is profitable to focus upon historical referencing because ultimately the histories of worlds (like world territory, world identity and world location among others) are themselves subject to contestation and interpretation and are thereby shaped by world members' accounts.

We must be precise regarding the remit and nature of the analysis outlined here. SWT is primarily constructionist and as such it stresses the partial and contextualised nature of all historical accounts. The analysis presented in this chapter acknowledges these points. Our concern is not to provide a definitive or comprehensive history of nursing and its relationship to other practices (CAM) and professions but instead to outline and reflect upon recourse to history employed by members of one sub-group set within the wider parent world of nursing. The presentations of history analysed in this chapter are firmly set within the conceptualisation of worlds and sub-worlds contesting both CAM/nursing integration and the wider historical location, essence and development of the nursing profession itself. As Strauss reminds us in his outline of a social world perspective, in addition to seeking out the histories of a world we should also 'question more properly . . . which histories – and whose histories – are we considering' (Strauss 1978: 228).

Thus in defining our key terms we are taking certain elements of parent terms (nostalgia and nostophobia) and combining them with insights from SWT in order to provide concepts appropriate to the specificity of nursing worlds and sub-worlds. *Nostalgic referencing is defined* as 'allusion to the past, grounded in a partial, contentious, arguably romanticised and necessarily constructed view of events; one that aims to legitimise current thoughts or actions of individuals, worlds or sub-worlds, and includes the re-discovery or re-deployment of all or some of a cited historical event or period.' We can conceptualise *nostophobic referencing* as the mirror of this: a negative interpretation of past events or periods, applied to underpin its rejection or removal from future action in favour of an identified alternative that is in keeping with specific objectives.

Method

We conducted a text analysis of papers published from within 'the nursing community' (see below) on CAM. The method was selected as it provided the most direct access to unsolicited public presentations. These were accounts produced for the public and professional consumption rather than for research purposes. Clearly, a substantial number of publications may contain one or more articles relevant to CAM nursing. It was therefore necessary to select journals on which to focus. We sought journals that would be likely to publish relevant papers, would provide a variety of styles (refereed and non-refereed, specialist and general, and articles on trials, theory and policy), and would address a range of potential audiences (journals targeted at specialist, academic and general nurses). These concerns were coupled with the need to ensure that the number of texts produced by the search did not become so large as to compromise the capacity to conduct detailed analysis. The selection of four journals – *Complementary Therapies in Nursing and Midwifery, Journal of Advanced Nursing, Nursing Standard,* and *Nursing Times* – satisfied these requirements.

Keyword searches (*Complementary Therapies, Alternative Therapies, Complementary Medicine, Alternative Medicine*) were conducted using MEDLINE, AMED and BRITISH NURSING INDEX databases for articles published in the four journals between January 1995 and November 2000 (selected as a period of considerable activity on integration between CAM and nursing – House of Lords 2000). This database search was supplemented by a manual search. As specific journals during a specific period were being searched, we can be confident that few if any relevant articles were missed. These keywords were chosen to capture the range of titles often employed by writers and commentators when referring to CAM practices (Vickers 1993). The decision was taken not to include individual therapy titles (e.g. 'aromatherapy') as keywords due to the vast number of potential therapies (BMA 1993) and the problem of deciding exactly which therapies are to be included or excluded from the field (Saks 1992; Sharma 1992). The combined search identified 278 papers.

Selection criteria are a central concern in text analysis (Deacon et al. 1999). Our inclusion criteria for articles from the journals were: a focus upon or relevance to the UK (as the first work of its kind in the area it was felt to be important to establish context specific themes that could then be challenged in other settings world-wide rather than produce a superficial international analysis); discussion of CAM or CAM integration in nursing; and articles authored by nurses or others with professional nursing roles (e.g. nursing administrators, nursing academics, but excluding medics). This last criterion was important because of the theoretical perspective from which the study was approached. Our interest was with the presentation of CAM nursing from sub-worlds *within* the nursing community. The practical task of identifying appropriate authors was easily managed via reference to the author details accompanying journal papers. Employing the criteria outlined above eighty articles were identified for further analysis.

Themes and propositions were generated independently by the two authors (such researcher triangulation provides a strategy to improve analytical validity [Rice and Ezzy 1999]). Analysis began with a detailed and separate reading of all the articles to achieve familiarisation with them. The data was then coded and key themes, which might illuminate processes relating to the intersection of CAM and nursing, were identified. Each author then challenged the other's interpretations and pursued negative cases. Where new findings ran counter to interpretations revised propositions were established and tested.

Analysis

The following data illustrates how a particular view of the past is called upon by authors in their presentations of CAM nursing. This is evident both in relation to an interpretation of the 'true' meaning of nursing in broad historical context, and in more precise references to defining moments and a 'golden age', specifically in relation to the pivotal figure of Florence Nightingale.

Our analysis of the texts led to the need to distinguish between differing rhetorical forms. Consequently, we have delineated two (inter-related yet distinct) ways in which this recourse to history is operationalised. These are termed static/conceptual rhetorics and dynamic rhetorics. Static/conceptual rhetorics are geared towards establishing the historical affinity between nursing and CAM as an end in itself. Dynamic rhetorics share many of the same emphases but go further in that they are structured in such a way as to use 'evidence' in an action orientated manner: primarily to justify ever-closer integration, or to highlight ways in which existing structures and powerful actors therein work to prevent that. Examples of both forms (static = s, dynamic = d) are included in cited quotations.

CAM and the historical 'reality' of nursing

The attempt to establish both that there is a general, deeply ingrained, affinity between nursing (principles and practice) and CAM practice, and that an examination of the history of nursing practice lends support to this, are pivotal themes running through the analysed papers. In this opening section we highlight three features of taken-for-granted constructions of what nursing is, and has been, throughout history. Nostalgic and nostophobic interpretations are in evidence concerning the character of nursing and the structural location of its practice.

Caring in an increasingly rationalised world

Underpinning much of the discussion in the texts is a conceptualisation of nursing as above all else an essentially human activity, concerned to promote those values that have become increasingly marginalised in an ever more rationalised environment of health care; one in which medicalised treatment regimes have dominated at the expense of human contact. In line with the rhetorics employed by others in nursing in support of practices other than CAM (Wilson 2000) the historical task of nursing is seen, within the texts, as something very different from this technical fix. There is a dual approach to historical referencing: a nostalgia for care orientated human level practice, and a nostophobia about more recent institutional arrangements.

Many of the developments of recent history are an anathema to the presentations of appropriate practice offered in the texts. There are many references to the desirability of 'getting back' to a style of practice associated with an earlier period in nursing:

> For nurses in particular, incorporating a complementary therapy into their practice has allowed many to get back to what they see as real nursing, that is hands-on, individualised care
>
> (70, d)

Elsewhere 'traditional' (despite the potential for confusion this term is widely used in the texts to refer to technically orientated, medically dominated, practice) nursing practice is contrasted with that of CAM. Nostophobic referencing of an era dominated by restrictive hierarchical structures and professional relations is introduced to underline the practice level impediments to integration within a 'traditional' structure.

> Nursing as a profession is nothing if not bound by hierarchy, and it may be difficult where a nurse is expected to be subservient to her supervisors or medical colleagues with her traditional nursing hat on, but wishes to take full responsibility as a holistic CAM practitioner with her CAM hat on
>
> (41, d)

Here, medicine and some sections of the nursing community itself are associated with traditional nursing; CAM with 'non-traditional' nursing. This formulation draws our attention to the importance of both inter-professional demarcations, and intra-professional boundaries within nursing itself. These identified boundaries act as a powerful rhetorical resource that complements the historical referencing in the texts.

The theme of the contrast between 'traditional' practices and perspectives in nursing and 'non-traditional' CAM is continued elsewhere:

> The increasing acceptance of complementary therapies . . . is welcome. Will such nursing developments challenge traditional perceptions of nursing practice and the nurses role within the team?
>
> (32, d)

Other texts more explicitly encase the need for CAM integration within a presentation of contemporary health care and society as essentially alienating. Here we are seeing a conceptualisation of CAM nursing as something very much broader than an occupational practice. CAM nursing is presented as being located within a need to redress the historically recent tendency to the dehumanisation of society: a postmodern critique of the modernist tendency to reductionism.

> A 'paradigm shift' is in effect taking place, which sees nursing, as part of a 'postmodern era', moving away from traditional health-related practices towards a more enlightened era . . . such a change can be incorporated into our profession . . . providing a powerful force for change in order to 'humanise' the current system
>
> (33, d)

> Nursing as we all know, is not simply a way of 'doing' for the patient, it is equally, if not more importantly, a way of 'being' with the patient. This has always been so, things have not changed, but perhaps the need for this kind of nursing is increasing in a society that promotes individualism and survival of the fittest as its dominant ideology hallmarked by the detachment and distancing of the market economy of health. Perhaps this explains nurses' keenness to incorporate complementary therapies into their care, to return a little connectedness to nursing
>
> (1, d)

And this notion of one form of nursing practice as dehumanising and distanced from patients is elsewhere directly compared with the development of CAM in more 'holistic' and 'innovative' nursing:

Technologically induced distancing of nurses from patients, a result of the rapid development of high technology in settings such as intensive care, has led nurses to include hands-on complementary therapies, such as aromatherapy, massage, reflexology, and shiatsu in their work

(64, d)

While engaging in a positive nostalgic referencing for the 'true' nature of nursing – its innovative and patient-centred character and so on – there is a (perhaps necessary) rejection of those aspects of (generally more recent) practice that have acted to hinder the development of this ideal form of nursing practice. The nostophobic referencing of medically dominated practice is perhaps the essential companion to the nostalgic imagery.

Innovation and flexibility

Beyond these broad, essentially conceptual, discussions of the place of CAM in the historical evolution of nursing, authors of texts drew out rather more practical dimensions of professional character and action, to support the authenticity of CAM in nursing. One example of this is the presentation of nursing as intrinsically innovative and flexible. The basis of the argument is that throughout history nursing has *repeatedly* incorporated techniques to extend the profession's boundaries. Given that change – be that the re-discovery of lost arts, the appropriation of new skills or whatever – is essential to the CAM nursing agenda, a partial or romanticised image of nursing on this issue clearly offers potential strategic benefit.

Nursing has a long tradition of borrowing techniques from a range of disciplines in order to increase its repertoire of interventions and enhance patient care

(72, s)

Nursing as a profession . . . *has always* been a leader in the evaluation and implementation of new treatment protocols which prove to be of benefit to the patient

(56, d; emphasis added)

If this case – of fundamental flexibility and innovation – can be successfully supported, it could prove very useful to advocates in two ways. First, the incorporation of CAM can be seen to be entirely in keeping with established professional practice. Second, this 'borrowing' of therapies provides the basis for a strengthening of nursing as a profession – by providing it with an increased range of therapeutic interventions. Both can be assumed to be beneficial when engaging in intra-professional debate.

The presentations of nursing as flexible and innovative are also directly contrasted with interpretations of medicine as historically restrictive upon, and controlling, nursing practice. Nurses' introduction of CAM is seen to provide a point of demarcation from medicine (Adams and Tovey 2001). Thus what is taken to be an essential element of nursing through the ages (innovation) facilitates the appropriation of CAM; this in turn provides the potential for success in 'the long struggle to establish epistemological demarcation from medicine' (Allen 2000: 327) that has been characteristic of nursing over recent years. In the following quotation attention centres upon the unequal power relations between the two professions which are seen to underlie the historical conflict between them:

> It is difficult for nurses to introduce complementary therapies into their practice without the permission of medical colleagues . . . This sort of dynamic is well documented in the literature and has frequently been the rock on which nursing innovations falter
>
> (45, d)

Once again the nostophobic allusion to an era of medical dominance is grounded in a belief that such structures are not just contrary to the principles of CAM nursing but are actively engaged in preventing its development. This dynamic – set within the historical relations between the two professions – is presented as an impediment, to not only the utilisation of CAM, but to the full expression of nursing innovation more broadly. Indeed, elsewhere the CAM debate is extended to embrace another core feature of medicine-nursing relations – gender. Here the barriers to an integration of different modes of healing are presented as essentially one and the same as those perpetuating the subjugation of nursing as a whole.

> Nurses, a largely female workforce, have been constrained by an imposed traditional view of healers as men that are, typically, medics or clerics . . . Any challenges will inevitably be met with a degree of scepticism, and on some cases, distrust
>
> (10, d)

Professional selflessness and the patient interest

Another feature of the image of nursing presented in the texts is of a profession historically shaped by a fundamental selflessness: a depiction of the profession's behaviour as being ultimately guided by client interests (see Lane Chapter 7 this collection for detailed discussion of the patient-centred approach with regard to midwifery). Indeed, as seen in a quote in the previous section, the 'borrowing' of therapies is characteristically presented as being geared towards the patient. This is imagery that has often been utilised to refer to CAM integration within nursing (UKCC 2000a) and also to define nursing practice and theory more generally (UKCC 2000b). Because it is central to professional ideology more broadly the ability to incorporate it is all the more important. The appropriation of the core rhetoric of client centredness serves to reinforce the authentic character of the affinity between CAM and nursing.

> A fundamental tenet of nursing practice . . . has always been to put the needs of the patient [first] . . . [T]he profession owes patients and their families the opportunity to utilise every resource available in order to accelerate the healing process
>
> (56, d)

What we see here moves beyond a static presentation of affinity. This is a good example of a dynamic rhetorical form. A nostalgic image of nursing – one in which the patient has *always* been put first (presumably beyond personal or professional self-interest, and again presumably in contradistinction to medicine) – is coupled with an expressed professional *duty* to patients and their families. This results in an *obligation* to embrace the widest range of therapeutic options, including, of course, CAM. In this case not only are the central tenets of nursing (through history) seen to be compatible with CAM utilisation, they actually demand it. A nostalgic interpretation of nursing is being called upon, but not as an end in itself. It is employed in an attempt to shape future practice.

In other texts the notion of patient-centred care (or patient-driven care) is called upon to frame more recent developments in nursing practice. A patient-centred approach to nursing is contrasted with task orientated care associated with earlier (medically dominated) times. Here the notion of patient-centred care is constructed in terms of tailoring therapeutics and nursing practice to the individual patient.

> A restructuring of nursing away from task orientated care towards primary nursing and the case approach . . . is facilitating an increase in nursing autonomy and in the provision of individualistic client care
>
> (28, d)

Another text draws upon similar imagery:

> Nursing appears to be at a cross-roads. Although not a new experience, the route taken will define the future of nursing. The first road leads to highly educated and respected practitioners, developing skills from medical colleagues, releasing them to make bigger and better medical

breakthroughs. The second route demands we challenge the contemporary pursuit of status and prestige to evolve the unique therapeutic patient-centred function of nursing

(55, d)

This quote draws heavily upon historical referencing both with the use of the word cross-roads (a break from the past) and also the notion of 'contemporary' circumstances. While embracing the ideology of nursing as motivated by patient-interest, nostophobic imagery is employed to implore a move away from recent approaches in nursing (dominated by concern with medically influenced approaches and focusing upon prestige and self-interest rather than patient centredness). It is argued that nursing needs to *get back* to patient-focused care (this is exemplified by the suggestion that the cross-roads now facing nursing 'is not a new experience'). Again we can see the parallel employment of nostalgic and nostophobic referencing. On the one hand the portrayal of recent nursing history evokes nostophobic imagery while, on the other hand, the very abandonment of this recent history is presented in nostalgic terms as hopefully revisiting some earlier golden era in the profession's development.

CAM nursing as historical reality

Thus, in the above we see the first evidence of the use of claims concerning the practical as well as the 'conceptual' historically grounded authenticity of CAM nursing. In certain texts this was taken a stage further: nurses themselves were presented as early pioneers of CAM. Here the suggestion is of nursing *returning* to a mode of holistic practice that has existed previously – at least within a section of the profession. In these terms CAM and nursing are historically bound as well as conceptually linked.

It is interesting that early moves towards the integration of certain healing therapies within health care was initiated by nurses . . . perhaps we share more in common with our ancestors than we thought

(manuscript 44, s)

The use of massage by nurses is not a new phenomenon. In 1895 a small group of nurses employed as 'medical rubbers' in London hospitals formed the Society of Trained Masseurs

(77, s)

We might see these examples as early illustrations of integrative practice: the combination of practices across orthodox and non-orthodox provision. Integrative practice is currently the subject of much practical experiment and theoretical discussion (Bettiens 1998; Hoffman 2001; Meines 1998).

It also frequently escapes problematisation. For instance, it is rarely asked what the boundaries are between integration, assimilation, appropriation; or, what the differences are between integration as the co-working of experts, versus integration as the combination of practices by an individual or single professional group. Indeed, despite the apparent enthusiasm of many advocates some evidence is beginning to emerge of how difficult it is to establish cross-profession and cross-sector integrative practice. It has been argued that many of these difficulties relate to inter-professional working and the varying conceptual frameworks of those involved (Coulter 2004). Where practices are appropriated and operationalised by an individual (person or group) such difficulties are of course diminished. And so there is theoretically much to be gained by orthodox professional groups following this route. By drawing on history, nurse advocates of CAM use are able to conceptualise appropriation/assimilation/integration (linguistic precision being of limited importance in this context) *by their own professional predecessors* as familiar to those with which they need to engage – colleagues in contemporary nursing. That familiarity acts to authenticate the controversial. And as noted earlier the viability of sub-worlds is dependent upon that capacity to authenticate.

History and the legitimisation of therapies

History is also called in to play in the texts during discussion of the nature of the (complementary) therapies themselves. This should be seen within the context of one widely recognised weakness of CAM: the lack of 'scientific' evidence to support its use (House of Lords 2000). If evidence cannot be called on to support the validity of practice, what can? Longevity could certainly be used to this effect. In the same way as familiarity has been seen to serve a clear purpose elsewhere in this chapter, so too it is useful in relation to the therapies used.

> Providing healing in an orthodox setting raises issues. One is to do with . . . what is erroneously described as the new-age movement . . . a surprising misnomer because such approaches are based on very ancient ideas and practices and are not new at all
>
> (40, d)

In the above example this is operationalised through a distancing from the language of new age, with its overtones of the contemporary, and perhaps more importantly, of fad or fashion. External validation may be achieved through an identification with 'ancient' arts; therapies that have survived modernist philosophy and (medical) practice. The generalised nostalgia for a more 'human' era is temporally extended.

CAM and Florence Nightingale: appropriating the defining icon

Perhaps the single most interesting historical theme to be drawn from the texts is the use of Florence Nightingale both to underpin the conceptual affinity between nursing and CAM, and to provide a legitimacy to the case for ongoing incorporation. References to Nightingale are interesting in the way in which they can be seen to share some of the emphases of the issues detailed above. While the specific content of presentations vary, in each case a level of consistency is evident. We see constant reference to how CAM's reliance on the 'natural' is matched by a similar emphasis by Nightingale. Thus we are seeing a similar process of familiarisation to that introduced earlier; this time directly focused on claims about nineteenth-century nursing practice. Now the potential for authentication is enhanced by being able to draw on the defining icon of nursing for evidence.

> Nurses and midwives can bring nature more consciously into clinical environments in many ways. In a basic way this is done by following Florence Nightingale's directives concerning pure air and water, light, cleanliness, and noise . . . [I]ncorporating complementary therapies provided by nature into care with patients . . . is a way of bringing a more conscious partnership with nature into clinical practice
>
> (12, d)

Similarly, the nostalgic referencing of Nightingale serves to act on another of the broader themes found in the writing – the need to counter-act charges of newness, fad and fashion. For here while the therapies may not be claimed to have been used by Nightingale, they have been presented as being 'provided by nature' – the very force said to be at the heart of Nightingale's approach to nursing.

Other texts show a similar propensity to draw on the theme of nature and Nightingale to underpin conceptual affinity and CAM utilisation. As with the opening quote, the following are clearly dynamic rhetorics. This is no mere exercise in the history of nursing. The incorporation of nostalgic imagery is explicitly concerned with establishing the basis for the inclusion of CAM into practice.

> Certainly Nightingale's [definition of nursing], 'to put the patient in the best condition for nature to act upon him (sic)', is indication for the inclusion of complementary therapies into nursing care
>
> (39, d)

> Many complementary therapies are based on the principle that disease is caused by an imbalance in a person's energy . . . and that re-establishing a balance will help people heal themselves. Nightingale believed that the

goal of nursing was to 'put the patient into the best condition for nature to act upon him (sic)', so nursing could be said to share many of the same values and beliefs as the complementary therapies that could be incorporated into nursing care

(72, d)

In the reclaiming of Nightingale CAM orientated writers are providing a new take on a strategy previously employed by other nursing sub-groups in professional debates surrounding nursing's role and identity (Duff 1998; McDonald 1998; Wheeler et al. 1999). However, it is worth highlighting something of a contradiction (or at least a point of potential contestation) in the use of Nightingale. This use is occurring at a time when some within the profession are distancing themselves from her image in an attempt to assemble a culturally dynamic base to modern nursing (Hallam 2000). Thus, while often presenting themselves as the forerunners of an innovative and daring expansion of nursing boundaries, on this dimension at least, CAM nursing may be seen to be operationalising an inherent conservatism in its attempt to authenticate therapies.

Discussion

In this chapter we have presented findings from an exploratory study of the content of articles produced by writers within nursing on the theme of the integration of CAM and nursing. The work is exploratory on two levels. First, this is the first time such nursing texts on CAM have been the subject of analysis. Second, the core concepts of nostalgic and nostophobic referencing are new. They are developed here specifically in relation to the CAM/nursing arena. Nostalgia and nostophobia are likely to fit into a complex pattern of processes through which the mainstreaming of CAM is pursued – although that is an issue to be resolved by further research.

We set two inter-related aims for the chapter. The first was to argue for a preliminary position (i.e. one explicitly open to modification following further work), that *nostalgia* and *nostophobia* are being used as identifiable rhetorical strategies by advocates of CAM/nursing integration; and that this is occurring in order to facilitate that integration and so promote a particular conception of what nursing should be. The second was to suggest the potential utility of the concepts of nostalgic and nostophobic referencing for the emerging sociology of CAM and nursing. These concepts result from the development and fusion of existing literature on nostalgia and nostophobia, with insights from social worlds theory. Central to the definition of *nostalgic referencing* is the partial, at times romanticised, interpretation of the past called upon to meet current needs of worlds or sub-worlds. Nostophobic referencing is recourse to a negative interpretation of a given historical period or practice for similar reasons. As we have seen these two forms of historical referencing are frequently employed in combination. This feature adds strength to the rhetorical presentations in the texts. A flexibility is employed as different elements are drawn upon, emphasised and appropriated to authenticate CAM integration to the nursing setting.

We have seen throughout the chapter how nostalgic and nostophobic referencing are used to support a case for increasing CAM integration. This was evident whether the focus was on broad components of nursing history (such as patient centredness) or on a quite specific event (the writings of Florence Nightingale), identifiable in time. And, crucially, these rhetorics took two forms: ones in which the author set out to establish conceptual or practical affinity (static) and ones in which texts moved beyond this to explicitly address how nostalgic imagery provides the basis for action, the basis of further integration (dynamic).

Thus nostalgic and nostophobic references were employed across a range of issues and in each case the interpretation of history fed a wider agenda – CAM integration. For instance, references to Florence Nightingale were packaged in the texts in a highly selective manner. The presentation of Nightingale is such that the bases of her philosophy and what are often taken to constitute the broad principles of CAM (supporting nature's capacity for healing) are almost inter-changeable. We are presented with a nostalgic image of nursing's defining icon. This explicit linkage between them makes sense as part of a strategy of authenticating the currently contentious or marginalised. Indeed in certain cases it was quite explicit in the texts that the authority provided by this interpretation of Nightingale establishes a clear impetus to integration.

It is interesting to compare the nostalgic recall of Nightingale in the texts with those features of a nostalgic discourse, appropriate to the macro level, identified by Turner (1987). If we accept Turner's list as an ideal type of nostalgia, seek to establish a (necessarily simplified) ideal type of the conceptual underpinnings of the 'CAM critique' of medicine and late modern society and draw out themes emanating from the CAM/nursing sub-world in this study, we can see strong overlap, even inter-changeability. The elements of: a sense of historical decline and a move away from a golden age of homefulness; the loss of personal wholeness; the sense of individuals operating in an ever more rationalised world, devoid of genuine social relationships; and the loss of emotional spontaneity, personal authenticity and simplicity are fundamental to each. Clearly, nostalgia (and its conceptual flip side – nostophobia) are evident features of these public presentations of the CAM/nursing sub-world.

Now if we acknowledge that nurses are using nostalgic and nostophobic referencing as strategies to authenticate the use of CAM, we are led on to the inevitable question of why? To begin to make sense of this we need to acknowledge, and return to, two important features of context. The first is that the future character of nursing remains contested. Both externally, and crucially within nursing, there is debate about the nature of nursing, its responsibilities, its roles, and of course, the place of CAM within it. The second point relates closely to this. It is that the authors of the texts presented here should not be seen to represent nursing. In so far as they can be taken to represent any unified grouping, they can be combined as advocates of CAM/nursing integration. We can draw on the fundamental building blocks of SWT to help clarify things here. These two points together mean that not only can we see that these advocates occupy a sub-world of nursing, but that in order for that sub-world to be successful, they need to engage in processes of *persuasion*. As SWT explains, rhetorics should not be seen as purely descriptive but also as attempts to move an audience – they ultimately act to persuade others of the presentations and arguments as set out by the social world and its members (Clarke 1990). For if the model of nursing with CAM as a central component does not succeed, by definition other models in which CAM plays a less significant part will predominate. While there is much to learn about the actual processes through which *nostalgic and nostophobic referencing* become activated, the extent to which it makes sense as a strategy is rather clearer.

In focusing on both *nostalgic and nostophobic referencing* as something specific – as potentially useful conceptual tools to progress the sociology of CAM and nursing – we would argue that it is through the fusion and development of two distinct sets of writings – those on nostalgia and those on SWT – that the distinctive contribution of the concepts can be brought into focus. For in taking this route we are able to incorporate many of the fundamental dimensions of nostalgia and nostophobia across contexts, embrace a recognition of their active character and their persuasive purpose; and, go on to fuse this with the issues, constraints and possibilities that are peculiar to the social world of nursing, and more importantly, to the sub-world of CAM nursing, and their agenda of persuasion in the context of competing rhetorics. An understanding of how contemporary action is framed by historical referencing will form a necessary part of generating understanding across the range of research priority areas.

References

Abel, E. (1986) The hospice movement: institutionalising innovation. *International Journal of Health Services* 16(1): 71–85.

Adams, J. (2001) Direct integrative practice, time constraints and reactive strategy: an examination of GP therapists' perceptions of their complementary medicine. *Journal of Management in Medicine* 15(4): 312–23.

Adams, J. and Tovey, P. (2001) Nurses' use of professional distancing in the appropriation of CAM. *Complementary Therapies in Medicine* 9(3): 136–40.

Allen, D. (2000) Doing occupational demarcation: the 'boundary-work' of nurse managers in a district general hospital. *Journal of Contemporary Ethnography* 29(3): 326–56.

Bartholomew, R. E. and Likely, M. (1998) Subsidising Australian pseudoscience: is iridology complementary medicine or witch doctoring? *Australian and New Zealand Journal of Public Health* 22(1): 163–4.

Barton, T. D. (1999) The nurse practitioner: redefining occupational boundaries? *International Journal of Nursing Studies* 36(1): 57–63.

Bettiens, R. (1998) Integrating complementary therapies in mainstream care. *Australian Nursing Journal* 6(3): 33.

BMA (British Medical Association) (1993) *Complementary Medicine: New Approaches to Good Practice.* Oxford: Oxford University Press.

Clarke, A. (1990) A social worlds research adventure. In Cozzens, S. and Gieryn, T. (eds) *Theories of Science in Society.* Bloomington, IN: Indiana University Press, pp. 23–50.

Clarke, A. (1991) Social worlds/Arenas theory as organizational theory. In Maines, D. (ed.) *Social Orgsanization and Social Processes.* New York: Aldine de Gruyter, pp. 119–58.

Coulter, I. (2004) Integration and paradigm clash: the practical difficulties of integrating two contradictory paradigms. In Tovey, P., Easthope, G. and Adams, J. (eds) *The Mainstreaming of Complementary and Alternative Medicine: Studies in Social Context.* London and New York: Routledge, pp. 103–22.

Davis, F. (1979) *Yearning for Yesterday: A Sociology of Nostalgia.* New York: Free Press.

Deacon, D., Pickering, M., Golding, P. and Murdock, G. (1999) *Researching Communications: A Practical Guide to Methods in Media and Cultural Analysis.* London: Arnold.

Dew, K. (2000) Deviant insiders: medical acupuncturists in New Zealand. *Social Science & Medicine* 50(12): 1785–95.

Duff, E. (1998) Florence Nightingale: basing care on evidence. *RCM Midwives Journal* 1(6): 192–3.

Federspil, G. and Vettor, R. (2000) Can scientific medicine incorporate alternative medicine? *Journal of Alternative and Complementary Medicine* 6(3): 241–4.

Fox-Young, S. (1998) Nurses and complementary therapies. *Australian Nursing Journal* 5(9): 29.

Gabriel, Y. (1993) Organisational nostalgia – reflections on a golden age. In Fineman, S. (ed.) *Emotion in Organisations.* London: Sage, pp. 118–41.

Gilbert, N. and Mulkay, M. (1984) *Opening Pandora's Box: A Sociological Analysis of Scientists' Discourse.* Cambridge: Cambridge University Press.

Giuffe, M. (1997) Science, bad science and pseudoscience. *Journal of Perianesthesia Nursing* 12(6): 434–8.

Hall, B. and Allan, J. (1994) Self in relocation: a prolegomenon for holistic nursing. *Nursing Outlook* 42: 110–16.

Hallam, J. (2000) *Nursing the Image: Media, Image and Professional Identity.* London: Routledge.

Hisama, K. (1996) Florence Nightingale's influence on the development and professionalisation of modern nursing in Japan. *Nursing Outlook* 44(6): 284–8.

Hoffman, C. (2001) Integrated medicine conference report: can alternative medicine be integrated into mainstream care? *Complementary Therapies in Nursing and Midwifery* 7(2): 110–14.

House of Lords (2000) *Complementary and Alternative Medicine*. London: HMSO.

Kerr, A., Cunningham-Burley, S. and Amos, A. (1997) The new genetics: professionals' discursive boundaries. *The Sociological Review* 45(2): 279–303.

Levin, S. (1996) Alternative medicine: a doctor's perspective. *South African Medical Journal* 86: 183–4.

Lomsky-Feder, E. and Rapoport, T. (2000) Visit, separation and deconstructing nostalgia: Russian students travel to their old home. *Journal of Contemporary Ethnography* 29(1): 32–57.

Lupton, D. (2000) The heart of the meal: food preferences and habits among rural Australian couples. *Sociology of Health and Illness* 22(1): 94–109.

McDonald, L. (1998) Florence Nightingale: passionate statistician. *Journal of Holistic Nursing* 16(2): 267–77.

Meines, B. (1998) Should alternative treatment be integrated into mainstream medicine? *Nursing Forum* 33(2): 11–17.

Mukta, P., and Hardiman, D. (2000) The political ecology of nostalgia. *Capitalism, Nature and Socialism* 11(1): 113–33.

Opie, A. (1997) Thinking teams, thinking clients: issues of discourse and representation in the work of health care teams. *Sociology of Health and Illness* 19(3): 259–80.

Rayner, L. and Easthope, G. (2001) Postmodern consumption and alternative medications. *Journal of Sociology* 37: 156–78.

RCNA (Royal College of Nursing Australia) (1997) *Position Statement, Complementary Therapies in Nursing*. Canberra: RCNA.

Rice, P. and Ezzy, D. (1999) *Qualitative Research Methods: A Health Focus*. Oxford: Oxford University Press.

Rinker, S. (2000) The real challenge: lessons from obstetric nursing history. *Journal of Obstetric, Gynecologic, and Neonatal Nursing* 29(1): 100–6.

Salmore, R. (1998) Our heritage: a history of gastroenterology and gastroenterology nursing. *Gastroenterology Nursing* 21(2): 40–3.

Saks, M. (1992) The paradox of incorporation: acupuncture and the medical profession in modern Britain. In Saks, M. (ed.) *Alternative Medicine in Britain*. Oxford: Clarendon Press, pp. 183–200.

Saks, M. (1995) *Professions and the Public Interest*. London: Routledge.

Sharma, U. (1992) *Complementary Medicine Today: Practitioners and Patients*. London: Routledge.

Shibutani, T. (1955) Reference groups as perspectives. *American Journal of Sociology* 60: 562–8.

Siahpush, M. (1999) A critical review of the sociology of alternative medicine: research on users, practitioners and the orthodoxy. *Health* 4(2): 159–78.

Snyder, M. and Lindquist, R. (2001) Issues in complementary therapies: How we got to where we are. *Online Journal of Issues in Nursing* 6(2): manuscript number 1.

Strangleman, T. (1999) The nostalgia of organisations and the organisation of nostalgia: past and present in the contemporary railway industry. *Sociology* 33(4): 725–46.

Strauss, A. (1978) A social world perspective. *Studies in Symbolic Interaction* 1: 199–228.

Strauss, A. (1982) Social worlds and legitimation processes. *Studies in Symbolic Interaction* 4: 171–90.

Tovey, P. (1997) Contingent legitimacy: UK alternative practitioners and intersectoral acceptance. *Social Science & Medicine* 45(7): 1129–33.

Tovey, P. and Adams, J. (2001) Primary care as intersecting social worlds. *Social Science & Medicine* 52: 695–706.

Tovey, P. and Adams, J. (2002) Towards a sociology of CAM and nursing. *Complementary Therapies in Nursing and Midwifery* 8: 12–16.

Turner, B. (1987) A note on nostalgia. *Theory, Culture and Society* 4(1): 147–56.

UKCC (United Kingdom Central Council for Nursing, Midwifery and Health) (1992) *The Scope of Professional Practice*. London: UKCC.

UKCC (United Kingdom Central Council for Nursing, Midwifery and Health) (2000a) *Perceptions of the Scope of Professional Practice*. London: UKCC.

UKCC (United Kingdom Central Council for Nursing, Midwifery and Health) (2000b) *Position Statement on Complementary Therapies*. London: UKCC.

Unruh, D. (1980) The nature of social worlds. *Pacific Sociological Review* 23: 271–96.

Vickers, A. (1993) *Complementary Medicine and Disability*. London: Chapman and Hall.

Watson, J. (1998) Florence Nightingale and the enduring legacy of transpersonal human caring. *Journal of Holistic Nursing* 16(2): 292–4.

Wheeler, W., Spinks, M. and Attewell, A. (1999) Florence: death of an icon? *Nursing Times* 95(19): 24–6.

Wilson, H. (2000) The end of Florence Nightingale. *American Journal of Nursing* 100(7): 24.

Woolley, M. (1999) Beyond simulation: production and the nostalgia Industry. *SSSP.Net* 2(1), September.

Chapter 5

CAM, nursing and the meanings of care

Kahryn Hughes

Introduction

The ever-increasing integration and expansion of complementary and alternative medicine (CAM) within nursing (Tovey and Adams 2002) has given rise to questions about the meanings of CAM for nurses. This chapter will examine the place of CAM within nursing and the notions of 'care' and 'holism' upon which CAM integration depends. While meanings of care and holism vary within and across professions (Kaptchuk 1996; Cassidy 1998), these meanings are used to hold off and differentiate both individual identity, and professional boundaries (also see Shuval and Gross Chapter 6 this collection). Simultaneously, the hinge of 'care' invoked by the participants in the samples drawn upon for this chapter serves to integrate the often intrinsically contradictory health belief models underpinning allopathic medicine and CAM. Through building on definitions of *care*, what it should be, what it should address, who provides the care, and how it should be provided (Wilson 2000), nurses erase potential disjunctions and opposition between the contradictory health belief models of allopathic medicine and CAM in the context of care provision. Debates about (CAM) nursing care speak closely to sociological debates about the ethics of care more generally, and this chapter will consider the opportunities for critical engagement these two growing literatures offer each other.

Background of the sample

The data drawn upon for this chapter comes from two separate studies. The first study was designed to monitor the emerging outcomes of packages of CAM care and treatment provided for common mental health problems with a view to subsequently developing a holistic outcomes measure (Long et al. 2000). The second, separate, study was designed to identify nurses' core elements of affective and instrumental nursing care (Hughes and Forster 2002).

The first (CAM) study involved in-depth interviews with complementary therapists delivering the packages of care employed both within the National Health Services (NHS) (general practitioners [GPs], nurses, physiotherapists) and external to the NHS, and with their patients. CAM within the NHS included reflexology, acupuncture and aromatherapy. CAM commissioned by the NHS (hereafter referred to as private practitioners) included homeopathy, yoga therapy, massage therapy including ayurvedic massage, reflexology and aromatherapy. Some practitioners (NHS and private) used a range of therapies (see Long et al. 2000). These interviews aimed to explore perceptions of health and healing and the meanings of CAM for CAM practitioners, with specific reference to the health care setting in which they delivered their care. Broad themes emerging from the data, using simple content analysis, were then taken to a series of focus groups with all practitioners in order to 'map out' concepts such as 'holism' and 'holistic practice'. Such concepts were interrogated both in terms of what they covered/ described, and in terms of how their meanings shaped and challenged health care practices (particularly in NHS settings). The interviews used from this study for this chapter are with nurses using CAM in the NHS, a midwife/ nurse using CAM privately, and also interviews with GPs using CAM. The latter are included as they provide interesting comparison with nurses; their ideas of 'holistic practice' often closely resemble those of nurses using CAM, which often directly contradicts nurses' perceptions of GP care and challenges core assumptions in the nursing and CAM literature underpinning attempts at professional distancing.

The first phase of the second (nursing care) study developed interviews with nurses and patients on one acute and one rehabilitation stroke ward, exploring their perceptions and experiences of what constituted nursing care, using an iterative interview process where analyses of early interviews informed and extended later interviews. In the second phase of the research, common themes emerging from simple content analysis of the interview data were translated into dimensions, or 'elements', of nursing care, which were used in repertory grid interviews (Beail 1985). These were with nurses (including health care assistants) who had been interviewed in order to establish how far these themes reflected what they felt they had said, and to interrogate more closely their understandings of the core concepts emerging through the interviews (e.g. nursing, care, holism). This methodology was chosen to generate self-contextualised sets of individual constructs, and so form a meaningful data set with which to interrogate meanings of nursing and nursing care. This study sought, therefore, to interrogate meanings underpinning nurses' health care practices. The data emerging from the nurses interviews (in-depth, repertory grid) will here be used to explore how nurses define nursing care; and how 'holism', a core concept for these nurses, is used to define nursing. Overall, then, this chapter draws on a diverse and sizeable range of data where the core aims of each study were very similar:

namely to explore meanings of care, whether nursing, clinical or CAM in the context of a range of different health care modalities.

Considering the 'lens' of care

The literature on care has four main themes, although much of the more sociological literature on the ethics of care focuses mainly on the first three (see Sevenhuijsen 1998; Williams 2001; Daly 2002; Tronto 1993). These themes are, first, that the lens of care is a means by which to interrogate and account for women's situation (Daly 2002; Ungerson 2000), and as a means by which actively to constitute unequal relations, demarcated through 'race' (Ahmad and Atkin 1996) and disability (Silvers 1995; Barnes 2002); second, to understand the inter-relatedness of human relations (Sevenhuijsen 1998) and, thereby, third, a means by which to critically engage with, and interrogate, normative frameworks underpinning welfare policies on care (Milewa et al. 1999; Daly 2002; Sevenhuijsen 2000; Williams 2001). Fourth, somewhat separate from this debate, 'care' in the health literature concerns questions around which (type/aspect/dimension of) care is effective and results in recovery; what models of care are there/should there be and how to implement these (e.g. Mantle 2001); and what negotiations are required around supporting (or diffusing) 'roles' in care, both formal and informal, in health care settings (Allen 2000; Daykin and Clarke 2000)?

Underlying the first three themes is the common aim of using 'care' as a lens by which to critically engage with the sociological project of understanding social relations. In this way, sociological work on the ethics of care provides a broad critical framework within which to engage with the fourth theme, which in this chapter concerns both the nature of nursing (paid work/care; caring), and more particularly the complexities and conflicts contingent on the ongoing endeavour within nursing to integrate CAM into practice. Additionally, the specific concern of 'human inter-relatedness' (Tronto 1993) both speaks to, and is articulated within, representations of care in the data and, as a consequence, offers an entirely appropriate level of analysis for the data from these two studies. Briefly, it allows us to move beyond a simply descriptive account of the types of care provided in different health care settings and to explore how particular discourses of care operate within and constitute particular relational configurations (Hughes 1999). Thus, the chapter will: first, explore the underlying philosophies of care presented by the participants in and across both studies; second, consider the dimensions of care from each study: and third, reflect on how the 'human interrelations' (Tronto 1993) constituted through these practices are articulated within the representations of care provided by the samples. The chapter will then conclude with some reflections on the additions this level of analysis brings to the debate.

Philosophies of care: 'holistic care'

Across both studies the notion of 'holistic care' was invoked to describe the type of care provided by non-CAM nurses in their attempts to characterise nursing care, and GPs and nurses engaged in the process of integrating CAM into their care-giving practices. Across both samples, 'holistic care' was used as a descriptor of their particular care orientation as part of an ongoing process of differentiation. This process of differentiation serves several purposes. First, it operates as personal identity formation, for example, as having altered the practitioners' perceptions:

> it has made me think more about lots of other little things. As I said we all tend to go on about the spiritual, well I am not particularly a very spiritual person myself I must confess. So I do understand other peoples' views and opinions, but it has made me look at other things in their way of life such as their diet and their social activities. Not social from the point of view of do they live with good carers, do they have stairs to climb – which is what I looked at before, but about social interaction.
>
> (Aromatherapist, reflexologist, and physiotherapist, in-depth interview)[1]

Importantly, as Daly (2002) points out, practices of care operate on both an individual and a political level, and can be said to define a configuration of particular social and professional relationships (see Hughes 1999; Hughes forthcoming). Thus, second, this process of differentiation operates to distinguish between professions, whether nursing or clinical (Allen 2000; Mantle 2001; Norris 2001; Mizrachi et al. 2005):

> I think it is a bit different because especially with GPs, because they haven't got the time to be totally holistic. Whereas if they have been given an half an hour, I know it is not long, but it is time for you to get to really know that patient. You do get to know them and they become friends of yours, so you do get to know them so it is more holistic than a ten-minute GP's appointment
>
> (Aromatherapist, practice nurse, in-depth interview)

or between professionals in the NHS and private CAM practitioners, to demonstrate the consequences of CAM integration in NHS nursing:

> I probably go where they perhaps fear to tread on the patients with quite bad arthritis. And I think that an independent Aromatherapist without a nurse training background might just stop there, they might not do it on those sort of patients . . . because of the complications I think.
>
> (Practice nurse, aromatherapist, in-depth interview)

And third, this process of differentiation is conversely invoked in order to erase potential differences between different health belief models by claiming similarities in philosophical orientation on the basis of practice:

> I have been looking at using the oils in foot baths as a preliminary to then going on and doing some of our physio techniques that we would do anyway. For instance, using an oil that might reduce muscle spasm prior to them doing some balance work or whatever . . . What I have tended to do, I have tried to incorporate it as one technique with physio techniques.
>
> (Aromatherapist, reflexologist, and physiotherapist, in-depth interview)

It is at the hinge of *care* that CAM and nursing are most clearly unified in the interviews across both studies. However, representations of practices of holistic care reflect the divide in the CAM literature and in debates regarding the ethics of care (Sevenhuijsen 1998; 2000). Simply, there is an ongoing tension between what is done and how it is seen, and what ought to be done and how it ought to be seen (e.g. Tronto 1993; Mantle 2001). Thus, what people think they ought to do does not necessarily reflect practice (Kim 1999). In the nursing study it emerged that nurses invoked a number of 'models' of nursing care to illustrate 'best practice'. Best practice was, they argued, fundamentally holistic in its approach both in terms of the 'complete care' patients received, and also in terms of the philosophical orientation of the care-giving activities which sought to address and meet patients' needs on an individual basis (Hughes and Forster 2002). However, it was not always possible to provide such care.

Q: So when you're talking about nursing care as holistic what do you mean by that?
A: By looking at total patient needs, working with their activities of daily living, looking at their physiological, psychological, social needs, and filling those roles, looking at the patient as a whole. So I look after them from their feeding perspective, from their hygiene, I would do all of it. But I don't do all of it, I may look after their social needs, but I wouldn't be able to feed them, you know. In theory I would, but in reality you can't do that so I distinguish between my role as a ward sister in that I organise a lot of things, patients I don't know particularly well, and I give care nursing care which I consider to be my real job.

(Senior Sister, acute ward, repertory grid interview)

This tension between intention to provide holistic care and the possibilities and constraints for, and on, such provision in the nursing study was matched by a tension in the CAM study around the worthiness of providing holistic care contingent on integrating CAM, some saying that it should be provided because it does what allopathic medicine cannot do, while others suggested it extends or adds to the care already provided (see also Adams and Tovey 2001).

An addition to this debate is provided in the sociological literature on care (Bashevkin 2000) where ideas of the ethics of care are invoked to challenge reductionist and individualistic notions of practices of care and, in doing so, to challenge reductionist notions of human relations. Specifically, it is claimed that using the lens of care to understand human relations illuminates our fundamental inter-dependency (Tronto 1993) – a claim which speaks directly to definitions of holism both in the literature (Griffin 1993) and in the data:

> Looking at the whole person, all aspects of that person. As I was saying about not just the physical side, emotional and spiritual side. The social side, their family, their way of life. All things that have a bearing on that person.
>
> (Aromatherapist, reflexologist, and physiotherapist,
> in-depth interview)

Thus, the concept of 'holistic care' calls into play notions of the fundamental inter-relatedness of human beings, not only locally, but globally. In this way, the challenge of 'holism' and 'holistic care' for allopathic medicine is that it demands a major reconsideration of health and illness, treatment and the medical encounter, of the rights and responsibilities of all interactants, and furthermore of individuals' roles in dealing with health and illness (Adams and Tovey 2001; Hughes 2004). The core conceptual features of holistic care in the data across both studies closely reflect those identified by Adams and Tovey (2001). In particular, CAM are understood to extend nurses' (and doctors') therapeutic repertoires; are holistic and extend nurses' existing care orientation; provide them with the opportunity to do more of what they're good at (touch, hands-on therapies, emotional caring); and allow them autonomy and expertise as care practitioners distinct from doctors and consultants (able to practise CAM that doctors don't know about). Clearly, discourses of holistic care operate to bring together nursing and CAM modalities. How, then, do specific dimensions of nursing care link in with those underpinning CAM care, and how far do practices of holistic care operate to challenge allopathic medicine in the ways outlined above?

The relationship between dimensions of CAM care and nursing care

Table 5.1 provides an overview of the wide range of grounded categories that emerged from the analyses of the CAM study interview data. Each

Table 5.1 Holism and holistic practice within complementary therapy (taken from Long et al. 2000)

Health	Healing	Illness	Therapy/Treatment
As perceived by the individual The individual's own responsibility for health and disease	Wanting to get well Empowering the process of self-healing Gaining control Getting in balance	Finding out the real problem Looking at the whole individual within his/her life and social context	Targets the individual Negotiated An ongoing process
Relationship of the therapist and user	*Individual responsibility*	*Encouraging movement and change*	
Working in partnership User is encouraged to talk and therapist to listen Trust Confidence and supportive therapist	Re-educating the body and self Developing coping strategies	Changing attitudes (to health) and behaviour (lifestyle) The healing process needs time to occur Learning for coping in the long term	

subsumes a range of shades of meaning and is linked to the others (Long et al. 2000).

Building on the thematic analyses of the interviews and using focus groups with participants to check for comprehensiveness and consistency, the CAM study sought to extend the range of dimensions of holistic care that are currently included on existing outcomes measures such as the SF36. As a result four broad areas of holistic practice hitherto neglected were identified: (1) aspects of the relationship between the CAM practitioner and the CAM user (as a partnership); (2) the process of uncovering the nature of the condition (to identify the hidden condition and underlying cause); (3) elements surrounding the healing process and the individual's role therein (learning, educating, developing); and, (4) the role of time and change within this (the need for measurement over a sufficiently long period of time) (Long et al. 2000: 29). These broad areas directly map onto the dimensions of holistic nursing care that emerged from the nurses' study.

Nursing care as holistic

Taken as a whole, nurses' perceptions of care were constituted through three core domains: the organisational, bureaucratic, and hierarchical context of the care provided; condition-specific nursing activities; and the nurses' philosophical orientation of and towards nursing care (Hughes and Forster 2002). While the first two domains have consequences for professional boundary demarcation and differentiation mentioned earlier these are dealt with more fully in other chapters in this collection and will only be touched upon briefly towards the end of this chapter. The bulk of the following sections will instead concentrate on the philosophical orientation of nursing care, how it relates to 'holistic care', and the consequences of this for critical engagement with the integration of CAM into nursing.

The interviews demonstrated ongoing negotiation between a range of definitions of 'nursing care', nurses grappling with how what they did could be described as 'nursing care'. These negotiations concerned caring as an emotional endeavour; basic care, hands-on and physical care to do with the body care of patients; care roles, such as acute care, palliative and rehabilitation care; emotional and psychological care as, to some extent, distinct from physical care; and nursing roles referring specifically to nurses' responsibilities and grades, which refers to tasks undertaken by nurses but do not necessarily fall into any of the foregoing definitions of care. In this way, care was identified as either 'direct' (hands-on) or 'indirect' (organisational activities), where nurses identified conflict between care (direct) and role (indirect). Significantly, contradictions between care and role were frequently, although only partially, resolved by describing the nursing approach as 'holistic' (see also Daykin and Clarke 2000). In effect, 'nursing' emerged as a process by which groups of events and practices were organised by the nurse according to overarching features (ward, shift, type of stroke, etc.), in order to form individual instances of 'care' unique to each patient. Therefore, it was not possible to talk about 'nursing care' as a set of uniform practices, or as something that could be clearly defined as any one or two things, but as a dynamic and complex interplay of activities underpinned by a set of philosophical and therapeutic beliefs, necessitating a particular (holistic) orientation of the nurse towards the patient (Hughes and Forster 2002).

Holistic nursing care emerged as, first, continuous, 24-hour care that nurses provide for patients (in contrast to the hour-a-day contact the physiotherapist or occupational therapist may have), where nurses are involved with the patient at every stage of their hospital stay.

> The nurses, well, we're caring for the patients on a daily basis and we're not just seeing them for an hour, here and there, for a quick visit like the doctors do, we help them with all the activities of daily living. We are there, obviously not 24 hours a day, but somebody is, it's 24 hours of care in nursing.
>
> (Primary nurse, rehabilitation ward, in-depth interview)

In addition, holistic nursing care referred to the comprehensive range of responsibilities the nurse has towards the patient, incorporating their individual physical needs, emotional and psychological needs, their family needs and relationships (including liaising between hostile relatives), and any social needs raised by the patient (e.g. arranging pet care). In this context, nursing care was described as 'all care' or 'total care'. Finally, holistic nursing care was reflected and based on distinct relational engagements with both the patient and their family/relatives/informal carers.

> . . . it involves everything. Even if it's ringing up somebody's erm grandchild because they're worried about them, you know. That is important for that patient and what's worrying them that day and needs dealing with and I think that's part of the care is to deal with anything that's worrying them, so it isn't just hands-on physical stuff, it's everything.
>
> (Staff nurse, rehabilitation ward, in-depth interview)

Across the sample, nurses stated that the *way* that they do nursing jobs is in itself 'treatment', e.g. rehabilitative, therapeutic; where emotional, physical, psychological and social care are inseparably blended.

> A lot of it's the ways in which you do things rather than the actual things that you do. And I certainly think it's very, very satisfying, to help people to help themselves and to return home, or to return to some sort of living, and the way in which we do that makes it more satisfying . . . [P]erhaps that's because the way in which we work is more intimate, more closer relationship wise.
>
> (Sister, rehabilitation ward, in-depth interview)

This philosophical and physical orientation is not only of the nurse towards the activities in which she/he engage in the care of patients but also includes how the nurse actively structures patients' physical and psychological orientation to their environment. This overall philosophical orientation was considered to characterise nursing care as holistic, provided 24 hours a day and involving monitoring patients' changing needs, be these physical or emotional. Nurses considered each patient as requiring individual treatment, yet each had formulated a generalisable therapeutic and philosophical orientation towards patients. This tension between the *individual* and the *general* was implicit in definitions of nursing as holistic, operating to define and separate nursing from other professions, particularly clinicians who were perceived as treating the general, i.e. prescribing standard treatments, and requesting standard tests and was articulated as a tension inherent in the nurse/patient relationship – a point that will be taken up later in this chapter.

Dimensions of holistic nursing care – bringing nursing and CAM together

Closer analysis of the dimensions of holistic care revealed that nurses' understandings of holism mapped directly, although not completely, onto those of private CAM practitioners, CAM nurses and GPs using CAM interviewed in the CAM study. These core dimensions included activities under each of the overarching categories summarised in Table 5.1 excepting the category of therapist/user relationship. This section will consider how the dimensions of holistic nursing care (if only in part) in Table 5.1 map onto those dimensions of CAM care and then, in a separate section, consider the therapist/user–nurse/patient relationship.

A core category of differentiation for nurses between themselves and other professions, especially clinicians, across both studies was that of defining health and illness. Non-CAM nurses understood themselves to utilise broader definitions of health within their holistic orientation than other professions; rather than as an absence of pathology, a definition they said was particularly used by clinicians, health blended into 'well-being' and in this way touched on all aspects of an individual's life. In this way, notions of health for nurses were individualised rather than standardised; health emerges from individuals' self-perception and within their personal expectations of ability in the context of their lives. For nurses using CAM there was no expressed disjunction between their CAM and nursing orientation towards the patient. Individual perceptions of health and well-being served as benchmarks of success of the treatment (how well does the patient feel; how much better?). Across both studies all nurses said that each person's condition was specific; that while patients may fall into similar medical categories, the variation between each patient was such to necessitate nurses orientating themselves towards patients on an individualised basis. This was directly articulated by nurses using CAM who stated that they treated the individual not the disease; non-CAM nurses stated their intention was to provide individual patient-centred care. In this way, across both groups 'holistic care' therefore varies for each patient, and is negotiated on the basis of individual need. In the ongoing process of negotiation around what the care should involve, nurses said they were more likely to 'pick up on things' (i.e. illness, worsening of the condition, emotional problems) than clinicians. Time, in terms of prolonged contact, enhanced their opportunity to spot things and, further, the consequence of prolonged contact led to intimacy which enabled them to spot changes in the patients' condition. For nurses using CAM this differed in that patients would themselves present both improvement and worsening in condition and that the process of CAM therapy was one which actively sought underlying causes of problems.

I think if somebody comes with a bad back and so you will treat the bad back and the doctors will probably just give them some pain relief or something. But getting down to it is quite often caused by stress and you help to treat stress and get them to talk about it, you help them relax and so it helps the bad back. Just looking at them as a whole person and finding out what is causing the problems.

(Aromatherapist, nurse, in-depth interview)

Also part of negotiations around what holistic care embraces, was nurses' perceptions of the patients' responsibility in 'getting themselves better'. Non-CAM nurses stated that there was no point in trying to help people get better if they weren't willing to make an effort themselves, particularly on the rehabilitation ward where they saw patients as having responsibilities in engaging with therapeutic processes.

Their mental attitude obviously makes a big difference. I mean we do get some patients that don't have any motivation, nothing can be done sometimes, some they fail and some they die because they've decided, they've made that decision that life's not worth living now and they won't do anything for themselves and in the end the patient's got to put work in themselves otherwise nothing does happen.

(Primary nurse, rehabilitation ward, in-depth interview)

This was echoed by nurses using CAM who blended this pragmatic notion of health and recovery consequent on patient engagement in therapy, and the broader CAM-based perception of health as a positive orientation towards one's life. As part of this, information provision emerged as a strategy whereby health could be encouraged, but was subsumed under the category of 'empowerment' by nurses not using CAM, where effective information provision educated the patient, enabling him/her to change existing behaviour and thereby reduce risk:

I think knowledge is so important to people for them to be allowed to ask questions, part of my role is to give them information in a way that would benefit them, not talking above their head, giving the information that they need and also allowing them to ask me questions. So I think it empowers them, it really does empower them, and I think it empowers the family as well.

(Sister, rehabilitation ward, in-depth interview)

Interestingly, even specialist nurses did not see information provision as necessarily condition specific; nurses not using CAM suggested that it was important that people understood how their lifestyles may have contributed to their condition. While this was framed in terms of health risk behaviour, nurses using CAM were more likely to talk about patients 'investing' in ill-health over a number of years. Differences between the two samples lay in the CAM nurses' perceptions of individual responsibility not only as something they had to take on in their future but also something they had to acknowledge from their past.

In this way, nurses using CAM brought distinctly unique perspectives on the process of healing as the body re-educating itself. While the nurses who didn't use CAM suggested that it was the body's natural capacity for healing, nurses using CAM were more specific about how the body learned through therapy. Across both studies, however, the value of time both in terms of duration of contact, and in terms of the body's need for longer duration of therapy and care were closely similar.

Therefore, the broad areas of nursing holistic care both map onto and diverge from those identified in the CAM study (see Table 5.1). First, the character of the relationship between nurses and patients varied significantly between the two studies (see below); second, similarity in the findings from both studies arose where processes of uncovering the nature of the condition (to identify the hidden condition and underlying cause) which transformed nurses from carers into diagnosticians revealed that diagnoses were based on different types of knowledge (intimacy, familiarity) than those drawn upon by clinicians in making their diagnoses; third, elements surrounding the healing process and the individual's role therein (learning, educating, developing) were similar, and were particularly significant in developing specialist nurses roles; and fourth, the role of time and change within this was crucial to notions of care and recovery, although this varied between acute and rehabilitation wards. Briefly, however, core to the nurses' understandings of nursing care as holistic was the character or dynamic of the relationship between nurse and patient as contingent on the intimacy of care provided, the comprehensiveness of that care, and the prolonged nature of their contact with patients. This contrasted with nurses who integrated CAM into their nursing, where the nurse/patient relationship did not subsume all other categories but was equally important as that of CAM knowledge and expertise, distinct from nursing knowledge (although drawing on it and blending with it) and the expertise of other professionals (individuals or groups). The following section considers how practices of care conceive of and constitute particular nurse-practitioner/patient relations.

Care as a medium for relationships

It's just getting to know one another on a personal level is the first thing, because if you don't do that you can't do anything else really. So that's the basic most important thing I think, and once a patient knows you and knows that you know them, and know something about them, they develop a trusting sort of relationship then, you can work on the hard work, you can start the hard work that's involved in rehab. And it is hard work.

(Primary nurse, rehabilitation ward, in-depth interview)

The nurse/patient relationship emerged as an essential precondition for care to occur, in terms of patients both understanding what their participation in their care ought to be, and in feeling able to ask nurses for care in the first place. However, nurses have been somewhat criticised for this orientation towards the nurse/patient relationship that draws on discourses of holistic care:

In the more mystical versions of nursing work, it is claimed that nurse–patient relationships have therapeutic value and are the means through which nurses assist patients in finding meaning in their illness experiences.

(Allen 2001: 390)

In the nursing study the nurse/patient relationship did indeed emerge as a contributing factor to the patient's recovery, although opinion on how this relationship was reflected in improved outcomes was divided. For some nurses, because the nursing care was holistic and therefore encompassed all the patients' needs, the composite effect of such total care resulted in therapeutic benefits. For other nurses, the nature of a positive nurse/patient relationship could have therapeutic value through increased sense of well-being in the patient; and that positive psychological care could be translated into improved physiology through biochemical (e.g. endorphin) changes in the patient. Nurses also felt the more time they invested in these relation-ships, the more informed the relatives were likely to be (although this had to be contextualised by the stage of the patient's stay, and the state of the patient's health). Therefore, rather than aiding patients seeking meaning in their illness experiences, as Allen suggests above, a key practice in this rela-tionship was to assist patients in finding meaning and understanding in their care and treatment. Non-CAM nurses felt that there were potential benefits to patients' emotional and psychological well-being resulting from understanding what was going on (as far as they were able), and on both wards there was a strong sense of promoting the patients' sense of indepen-dence through physical support, involvement of the patients in their own treatment, and increasing their sense of decision-making power through such involvement and through information provision. Patients were expected to participate in their recovery process and appreciate that being positive was central to the recovery process. This positive attitude was felt by nurses to stem from confidence in their care which in turn emerged from confidence in their nurses. Increased confidence could result in a reduc-tion in anxiety which could positively affect their sleep, their emotional state and, in a systemic way, their health. However, this also required nurses negotiating patients' expectations in order to address and possibly reduce depression and low emotional mood. In attempting to deal with cycles of depression by being positive about potential recovery through small goal-setting activities, the nurses felt there was a fine line between being hopeful and being realistic. On the one hand, patients need to know how much work they have to do, otherwise they might be tempted to lie back and do nothing. However, being too negative might encourage them to give up hope in which case they lie back and do nothing anyway. In this way, nurses felt they were involved in transmitting their own professional and personal philosophical and therapeutic orientations to patients as part of the positive emotional and psychological orientation of patients to their recovery. Thus, the nurses' understandings of healing and the patients' role in recovery echoes those in CAM philosophy (Hughes 2004) and in the CAM nurses' explanations of their relationships with patients.

> So what I'm doing in my group sessions I try and open people up to look at themselves, how they are and how they fit in the world, and what reactions they're getting so they can start and think it is important to know yourself from the neck down and the neck up, change things, change movements, change situations, change diet, and life will start to be different, and if you don't do that they're heading for a hospital bed.
> (Yoga therapist, massage therapist, midwife, nurse, in-depth interview)

Nurse/patient relationships were thus held to underpin potential for recovery for patients operating through physical, emotional, psychological, familial and social effects.

The importance of the nurse/patient relationship also raised the tension mentioned earlier. This lies between the necessity to develop a relationship with the patient in order that nursing care could happen at all, and so developing an individual relationship with each patient while, at the same time, personal, professional and organisational constraints mitigate against these relationships becoming 'too personal' (see also Ungerson 1999). In the interviews, nurses described ongoing struggles they had around negotiating the degree of intimacy in their relationships with patients. The nurses stated that patient encounters involved negotiations around the character of a nurse/patient relationship which would provide the conditions wherein 'nursing' could occur. In this way, care was often conflated with caring, i.e. emotional investment on the part of both nurse and patient, where 'caring' comes into conflict with 'work'. For nurses using CAM, however, this conflation was sometimes described as normal and part of the thera-peutic process. For both non-CAM nurses and CAM nurses, however, holistic care-as-work was invoked in the process of professional boundary-setting; and this is one of the main areas of perceived differential success between non-CAM nurses and nurses engaged with integrating CAM into their nursing practice.

Some of the main differences

A central difference between nurses using CAM and nurses who did not use CAM lay in their descriptions of their autonomy as care practitioners. While non-CAM nurses subsumed every dimension of holistic care into the category of this relationship in which all care was made possible, organisational constraints impinged on the nurse's ability to provide holistic care, which often emerged as an aspiration and not necessarily the reality of the nurse's practice. However, nurses using CAM described their care practices as different. First, the techniques they are able to use; second, changing their approach to the patient:

Q: Do you feel that you have to change your approach when you are doing aromatherapy?
A: Definitely. Well in a way yes, you have to be approachable to the patient at all times. But most of these patients that we do aromatherapy on they are quite stressed and tense and they are concerned, so we slow down. You have to slow down your approach you can't be all brusque and businesslike. We play soft music and turn the lights down and generally slow down for half an hour, but then your brain has got to speed up again when you walk out of the door because there is somebody waiting for something else completely different.
Q: So what it is to be a practice nurse?
A: You have to have an alert brain to start with, but at my age it's not always as alert as it should be anyway! So you have to make sure you give the right injections and you are doing the right thing. So you have to be on the ball whereas five minutes ago you have just turned off gently massaging somebody's back with oils that send you to sleep.
(Aromatherapist, practice nurse, in-depth interview)

And third, the differences between the health belief models and subsequent interventions from both allopathic medicine and CAM:

I would see the health service as having three points of action, to give drugs, to use surgery, or chemicals, such as radiotherapy, and obviously the physiotherapy around it to complement what they're doing. I see health service, not so much as invasive, it is invasive, drugs are invasive internally, and it's just a set of principles in the health service to deal with each individual case, most of it's based on drug therapy as I see it . . . I see complementary as a different approach, it may take longer, and take a more roundabout way, but people open up to it and once we can get them open and understanding and looking at their life differently and changing their lifestyles so that these things don't reoccur, we can help them with their initial problems and guide and direct them to ways that need not be so invasive and quite so long-term. . . . I think complementary therapies . . . try and get people to look at themselves, how they are, how they think, how things are going on in their lives, some simple changes could change their health and well-being enormously.

(Yoga therapist, massage therapist, midwife, nurse)

In the CAM study, it was noticeable that the actual process of providing CAM care contributed to the formulation of different relationships with clinicians (nurses were given their own patients), but also different working spaces. Where aromatherapy is being provided, it is important that the scent from oils does not spread throughout the whole care setting as they may be contraindicated for conditions other patients are attending with. Further, separate working spaces are essential for therapies requiring tranquillity. Additionally, nurses explained that they were asked for their own assessment of outcomes from the treatment; that because the condition was transformed through the therapy process (i.e. translated into the therapeutic vocabulary of the CAM practised by the nurse), so were criteria for success. Rather than sharing a patient, or providing care prescribed by a clinician in a piecemeal manner, nurses using CAM are able to bring to the nurse/patient encounter a complete therapeutic repertoire. Thus although non-CAM nursing care was constituted as holistic through the nurse/patient relationship, and simultaneously care shaped relationships and connections, the extent to which their care was holistic was additionally shaped by the patients' condition, the organisational setting, and multi-disciplinary team needs. Comparison between the two studies suggests CAM nurses are more able to resist organisational constraints than nurses who do not use CAM, because they bring to their work more than an additional therapeutic tool to add to their repertoire; CAM allows nurses to further differentiate professional boundaries and responsibilities, and form relationships differently than nurses who don't use CAM, because they have an additional expertise; knowledge that isn't immediately available to clinicians or allied professions.

Conclusion

From this discussion, meanings of CAM and nursing care can be and are reconciled through discourses of holism. In this way potential tensions between contradictory health belief models can be elided or erased. Holistic care is invoked in order to define existing practice, develop and differentiate between individual and professional identities, and understand and constitute practitioner/patient relations. While discourses of holistic care may successfully reconcile nursing and CAM, this is not a powerful enough resource for nurses pursuing more authority and autonomy in their working lives; particularly evidenced in the nursing study presented here in terms of the extent to which they are able to deliver the types of care to which they aspire. Organisational constraints impinge upon such autonomy, expressed through conflicts between 'role' and 'care' – activities involving the patient, versus activities involving the bureaucracies of the service and organisation. Conversely, nurses using CAM are not only able to hold individual clinics within hospital and primary care settings, they are also able to develop their therapeutic repertoire through the use of CAM; autonomy over workplace and care-giving settings; different relationships with patients. CAM skills, techniques and expertise provide the opportunity for increased authority. One implication of this is that, rather than a disparate series of events, CAM care should be considered as a process (Long et al. 2000) where treatment is understood to operate over more prolonged periods of time than that provided in acute or rehabilitation hospital settings. In this way, the integration of CAM into nursing clearly opens up political spaces in which ongoing negotiations around the provision of patients, of appropriate care settings, and longitudinal aspects of treatment must occur within and between professions. In contrast to CAM nurses, for non-CAM nurses, invoking discourses of holistic care is insufficient as a strategy for differentiation in the pursuit of greater autonomy and legitimacy.

Using the lens of care, then, as a level of analysis allows us to critically explore the areas where discourses of holism fail in endeavours of professional boundary maintenance. Political spaces that are created through the ongoing integration of CAM which builds on, and extends, existing notions of holistic care while simultaneously erasing potential conflicts between underlying health belief models of allopathic medicine and CAM can be described. Using care as a lens by which to understand how potentially competing health belief models are reconciled between allopathic medicine and CAM, also provides the opportunity to explore the normative frameworks underpinning 'holistic' approaches to care. To begin with, care becomes work, and in this way enters a political arena in which activities such as professional boundary-setting can be critically engaged with. Also, drawing on Williams (2001), whose representation of the value of using care as a lens by which to understand human relations, allows us to directly address political consequences of the philosophies underpinning CAM and modern nursing strategies. Thus, Williams argues, care is an activity that binds us all, either as givers or receivers at different stages of our lives; that through care we can learn core normative values for citizenship, such as mutuality and responsibility; that inter-dependence is seen as the basis of human interaction, and attributes moral worth to key positive dimensions of caring relationships, such as trust, dignity and bodily integrity; care requires time, and recognition of choices; and, care is not only personal, it is an issue of public and political concern.[2] In this way, Williams seeks to normalise responsibilities for giving care; an aspiration echoed in how nurses describe holistic care, and how CAM nurses describe their efforts in integrating CAM into conventional treatment settings.

However, the ethics of care debate also allows critical analyses of the power differentials and inequalities in these carer/cared-for relationships. Recognising the activities that are involved in the work of care, particularly when practitioners are seeking to provide holistic care, allows us to critically engage with the potential for 'professional boundaries to become porous' (Ungerson 1999: 595).

Also, in building on normative frameworks of mutuality both allopathic and CAM nursing espouse activities such as information provision, encouraging involvement and responsibility-taking in the process of self-care and recovery, encouraging a sense of empowerment, and translating CAM practitioner/patient relationships into partnerships. These are of concern, however, because they are predicated on relationships based on crucial power differentials between patient and professional. These differentials also include those of health, and therefore ability and can often be problematic in overly encouraging both engagement in and responsibility for both recovery and illness where this becomes counter-productive (Hughes 2004). Further, differentials in lay and professional knowledge, and inequalities arising from the geographical/spatial dislocation of the patient, particularly when in formal care settings, are again problematic and require ongoing critical engagement. Therefore, while meanings of holistic care converge around principles of equality and mutuality, it is essential that we acknowledge that these are principles for practice rather than *conditions* for practice.

Therefore, bringing together the ethics of care and CAM care literature illustrates how human (and especially caring) relations challenge and make clearer broader professional power relations and the sociological agenda for critically engaging with these philosophical and pragmatic developments consequent on the integration of CAM in nursing.

Notes

1 Although this participant is a reflexologist, she was part of a broader initiative to introduce packages of CAM through clinical, nursing and allied professions. As a non-clinician, her responses were very interesting in that they reflected precisely the same demarcation activities as those in the nurses' and GPs' interviews.

2 This is only a selection drawn from a longer list in Williams (2001).

References

Adams, J. and Tovey, P. (2001) Nurses' use of professional distancing in the appropriation of CAM: a text analysis. *Complementary Therapies in Medicine* 9: 136–40.

Ahmad, W. and Atkin, K. (eds) (1996) *'Race' and Community Care*. Buckingham: Open University Press.

Allen, D. (2000) Negotiating the role of expert carers on an adult hospital ward. *Sociology of Health and Illness* 22(2): 149–71.

Allen, D. (2001) Review Article: Nursing and sociology: an uneasy marriage? *Sociology of Health and Illness* 23(3): 386–96.

Barnes, C. (2002) Disability, user-controlled services – partnership or conflict? In Leathard, A. (ed.) *Interprofessional Collaboration*. London: Routledge, pp. 200–11.

Bashevkin, S. (ed.) (2000) *Women's Work is Never Done: Comparative Studies in Care-giving, Employment, and Social Policy Reform*. New York: Routledge.

Beail, N. (ed.) (1985) *Repertory Grid Technique and Personal Constructs: Applications in Clinical and Educational Settings*. London: Croom Helm.

Cassidy, C. M. (1998) Chinese medicine users in the United States Pan 11: preferred aspects of care. *Journal of Alternative and Complementary Medicine* 4: 189–202.

Daly, M. (2002) Care as a good for social policy. *Journal of Social Policy* 31(2): 251–70.

Daykin, N. and Clarke, B. (2000) 'They'll still get the bodily care': discourses of care and relationships between nurses and health care assistants in the NHS. *Sociology of Health and Illness* 22(3): 349–63.

Griffin, A. (1993) Holism in nursing: its meaning and value. *British Journal of Nursing* 2(6): 310–12.

Hughes, K. (1999) From Anorexia Nervosa to Anorexic: the process of subject constitution in the therapeutic encounter. PhD thesis, Department of Sociology and Social Policy, University of Leeds.

Hughes, K. (2004) Health as individual responsibility: possibilities and personal struggle. In Tovey, P., Easthope, G. and Adams, J. (eds) *The Mainstreaming of Complementary and Alternative Medicine Studies in Social Context*. London and New York: Routledge, pp. 21–46.

Hughes, K. (forthcoming) Migrating identities: the relational constitution of drug use and addiction. *The Sociology of Health and Illness*.

Hughes, K. and Forster, A. (2002) *Developing a Framework of Nurses' and Patients' Constructs of Nursing Care*. School of Healthcare Studies, University of Leeds.

Kaptchuk, T. (1996) Historical context of the concept of vitalism in complementary and alternative medicine. In Micozzi, M. (ed.) *Fundamentals of Complementary and Alternative Medicine*. New York: Churchill Livingstone, pp. 35–48.

Kim, H. S. (1999) Critical reflective inquiry for knowledge development in nursing practice. *Journal of Advanced Nursing* 29(5): 1205–12.

Long, A., Mercer, G. and Hughes, K. (2000) Developing a tool to measure holistic practice: a missing dimension in outcomes measurement within complementary therapies. *Complementary Therapies in Medicine* 8: 26–31.

Mantle, F. (2001) Complementary therapies and nursing models. *Complementary Therapies in Nursing and Midwifery* 7: 142–5.

Milewa, T., Valentine, J. and Calnan, M. (1999) Community participation and citizenship in British health care planning: narratives of power and involvement in the changing welfare state. *Sociology of Health and Illness* 21(4): 445–65.

Mizrachi, N., Shuval, J. and Gross, S. (2005) Boundary at work: alternative medicine in biomedical settings. *Sociology of Health and Illness* 27(1): 20–43.

Norris, P. (2001) How 'we' are different from 'them': occupational boundary maintenance in the treatment of musculo-skeletal problems. *Sociology of Health and Illness* 23(1): 24–43.

Ruddick, S. (1989) *Maternal Thinking: Towards a Politics of Peace.* Boston, MA: Beacon Press.

Sevenhuijsen, S. (1998) *Citizenship and the Ethics of Care: Feminist Considerations on Justice, Morality and Politics.* London: Routledge.

Sevenhuijsen, S. (2000) Normative concepts in Dutch policies on work and care. In Bashevkin, S. (ed.) *Women's Work is Never Done: Comparative Studies in Care-giving, Employment, and Social Policy Reform* 1–18.

Silvers, A. (1995) Reconciling equality to difference: caring (f)or justice for people with disabilities. *Hypatia* 10(1): 30–55.

Tovey, P. and Adams, J. (2002) Nostalgic and nostophobic referencing and the authentication of nurses' use of complementary therapies. *Social Science and Medicine* 56: 1469–80.

Tronto, J. C. (1993) *Moral Boundaries: A Political Argument for an Ethic of Care.* New York: Routledge.

Ungerson, C. (1999) Personal assistants and disabled people: an examination of a hybrid form of work and care. *Work, Employment and Society* 13(4): 583–600.

Ungerson, C. (2000) Thinking about the production and consumption of long-term care in Britain: does gender still matter? *Journal of Social Policy* 29(4): 623–43.

Williams, F. (2001) In and beyond New Labour: towards a new political ethics of care. *Critical Social Policy* 21(4): 467–93.

Wilson, H. (2000) The end of Florence Nightingale. *American Journal of Nursing* 100(7): 24.

Chapter 6

Nurses and midwives in alternative health care

Comparative processes of boundary re-configuration in Israel

Judith T. Shuval and Sky E. Gross

Introduction

This comparative study of nurses and midwives practising complementary and alternative medicine (CAM) is an additional link in our ongoing research concerning the co-habitation of biomedicine and alternative medicine in Israel. We have been interested in negotiative processes of boundary crossing which take place when alternative practitioners work within the organisational context of biomedical institutions (Mizrachi and Shuval 2005; Mizrachi et al. 2005; Shuval 2001; Shuval and Mizrachi 2004; Shuval et al. 2002).

The present chapter expands the context of our research by focusing on two groups of allied health professionals who utilise CAM practises. Like increasing numbers of physicians who practise CAM, the nurses and midwives under study are trained and experienced in mainstream biomedicine and have at some point in their careers opted to study and practise a variety of CAM skills. Their experiences in the processes of boundary crossing are analysed in terms of 'boundary work' as discussed by Gieryn (1999) and in the manner proposed by Allen (2000) to include practices utilised in the work context.

Following the view that professional practice is more likely to be pluralistic than monolithic, we are interested in meaningful evidence of such pluralism. Going beyond dualism, we will seek a variety of dimensions of differentiation within these professions (Hirschkorn and Bourgeault 2005). This leads to a focus on intra-professional issues which we will consider on two levels: within each of the two groups and then on a comparative basis, between them. Thus the chapter will focus on differences among nurses and among midwives. After spelling out the implications of each of these, we will present a comparison of the two sets of findings.

CAM in Israel

Over 20 forms of CAM are in widespread use in Israel. In 2003 it was esti-
mated that 8,800 persons were engaged in full- and part-time practice. While
much of CAM practice is in the private sector, the mainstream public sick
funds all maintain special clinics where members may obtain CAM services
and 30% of the hospitals maintain outpatient CAM clinics (Shuval and
Mizrachi 2004).

The most recent representative survey data concerning use of alternative
medicine in Israel is based on two samples of the Jewish urban population
aged 45–75 carried out in 1993 (n = 2,203) and in 2000 (n = 2,505)
(Shmueli and Shuval 2003; 2006).

In 1993; 6.1% of the population reported consulting with non-
conventional medical practitioners at least once during the previous year; in
2000, that proportion increased to 9.8%. Increases are observed in several
socio-demographic groups: women, younger people, persons having 12 or
more years of schooling, persons with higher economic status and residents
of large cities. Between 1993 and 2000, non-conventional medicine in Israel
turned from an infant industry into a mainstream health commodity
(Shmueli and Shuval 2003; 2006).

Nursing in Israel

In 2003 there were 53,381 nurses in Israel of whom 65.5% were registered
nurses while the remainder were trained as practical nurses. Until the mid-
1970s nursing training in Israel took place in diploma schools affiliated
with hospitals. In 1975 the first programme leading to a university degree
in nursing for high school graduates was established by the Hadassah
School of Nursing at the Hebrew University of Jerusalem. Subsequently
the other schools of nursing and several of the other allied health occupations up-graded their diploma schools to university level (Bergman 1986;
Zwanger 1988). In 2003, 1,394 persons received an academic degree in
nursing: 87% a bachelors degree, 12% an MA and 0.3% a PhD.

Since the establishment of the first university-level nursing school in 1975,
nursing education in Israel has sought to combine a scientific biomedical
model anchored in empiricism and evidence-based medicine with an orientation based on an understanding of the integration of mind and body, prevention and empowerment of patients, and health education. The curricula
were expanded to include concepts drawn from psychology, sociology, and
communications theory (Salvage 1992). However, despite some changes,
nurses' formal socialisation remains predominantly biomedical and for most
that medical anchor provides security, status and closure in their epistemological orientation such that they do not question the traditional axioms of
biomedicine.

Over the years, nursing in Israel has been increasingly differentiated into specialties and sub-specialties which are formally defined and characterised by post-basic training. Among the nursing specialties are intensive care, emergency room care, public health, neonatal health, geriatrics, nephrology, oncology and midwifery. Nurses are employed in a wide variety of health care settings including hospitals, community clinics, mother and child care centres, schools, day-care centres, geriatric and rehabilitation centres and other institutions.

The need to provide employment for large numbers of immigrant physicians has made the medical profession and health authorities reluctant to expand the nursing role to allocate them greater formal responsibility. In addition, the general conservatism of Israeli women is reflected in the widespread acceptance by nurses of physicians' authority and the preference of most to place personal family and child-rearing concerns above those of their work (Shuval and Anson 2000).

Until the 1950s, nursing in Israel was strongly anchored in the Nightingale tradition which highlighted skills associated with nurturance, devotion, caring, obedience and 'mothering'. As in most other Western countries, it occupied a subservient position with respect to the dominant medical profession highlighting dependence and lack of autonomy. After World War Two, when it became increasingly clear that there was a need to redefine the roles and functions of nursing, nurses began seeking advanced academic degrees, initiated their own research and increased their knowledge base and skills. In recent years there is a growing interest in more egalitarian relations between nurses and physicians as well as between nurses and their patients (Hojat et al. 2003).

The relation of feminism to nursing is ambiguous in Israel. The feminist movement developed later and more slowly in Israel than in most other developed societies. This has been attributed to the conservatism of major segments of the population: strong familism and traditional gender role differentiation within religious groups as well as first and second generation immigrants from traditional societies in Asia and North Africa. The centrality of the army and its predominantly masculine ethic have also contributed to widespread acceptance of the unequal status of the genders (Shuval and Anson 2000). There are small numbers of nurses who seek greater autonomy and less control. These nurses tend to be critical of the overly technical-rationalist orientation of contemporary biomedicine and its failure to adhere to a holistic, empathetic, patient-centred practice. At the same time, there is little overt identification among nurses with the overall values of the expanding feminist movement (Allen 2000; Glazer 2000; Hoffmann 1991; Johnson 1990).

Interest in CAM among nurses in Israel developed in the context of changing values and norms in the profession which parallel, in large measure, the changes in nursing in other societies. Nurses practising CAM at the start of the twenty-first century represent a small, marginal group among nurses in Israel. As in other developed societies, they have been influenced by increasing exposure to Eastern spirituality and to postmodern values which have raised penetrating questions about the ability of science and technology to provide answers to human problems including illness (Coburn and Willis 2000).

Midwifery in Israel

Midwifery in Israel is one of many areas of specialisation in nursing. Thus midwives are qualified nurses who have completed an additional 9-month course in midwifery. This course combines theory with clinical experience and includes supervision of the trainee in at least 50 births. It focuses on the obstetrical model of care. Successful completion of the course involves passing a government administered examination which provides the midwife with a licence to practise. In 2003; there were 1,427 licensed midwives in Israel. They constitute 11% of the nurses with specialised training and 2.7% of all the nurses.

There are about 150,000 births a year in Israel. Almost all take place in hospitals – a condition established by law in 1954 which entitles receipt of a government maternity grant (the approximate equivalent of $300 for a first birth and $100 for subsequent births). In 2003 there were 290 planned homebirths; it has been suggested that this number is growing (Tel-Oren 2000).

Most hospitals have a midwife working in a reception section of the delivery ward to check arrivals in the early stages of labour and to fill in her chart before she is admitted to the labour ward. After admission, most hospitals have separate labour rooms for each woman. The woman is placed in a bed, attached to a foetal monitor and an intravenous (IV) routine is started. Vaginal checks occur about every hour. When there is a 4–5 cm opening, the woman is encouraged to take an epidural. In 2003, 39% of the births received an epidural. The routine tasks of midwives include rupture of membranes, attachment of foetal monitoring, injection of IV fluids, and delivery in lithotomy position.

Growing interest of midwives in CAM may be seen by their enthusiastic participation in courses in CAM geared specifically for midwives. A number of these have been held in the past 5 years in 6 different hospitals, in some cases under the sponsorship of the hospital administration. Examination of the curriculum of an 108-hour course for midwives in alternative health care techniques (offered at an elite Jerusalem hospital in 2004) shows that the following subjects were presented by expert practitioners in each field: shiatsu, reflexology, imaging, natural childbirth, naturotherapy, Paula technique, reiki, touch therapy, aromatherapy, herbal medicine, Chinese pressure points and body movement during labour. Most emphasis was placed on reflexology, reiki, imaging and natural childbirth (over 10 hours of instruction for each). In the above hospital, the course was partially subsidised by the hospital and all midwives were encouraged to participate. At the same time, the chief midwife, who was herself enthusiastic about the course, was reluctant to publicise its existence overtly.

Data collection

The nature of the research dictated the use of qualitative methods to obtain in-depth information from a small number of persons who are directly involved in the delivery of health care. Thus the findings are based on a qualitative analysis of in-depth, narrative interviews with 15 nurses and 13 midwives in Israel all of whom are currently working or worked in the recent past in both biomedical and alternative health care settings.

In seeking to locate such persons, it quickly became apparent that there was no comprehensive list of such practitioners. Utilising informal sources of information and the snowball technique, we learned that they are located in a variety of health care institutions, often work in multiple settings and may practise more than one form of alternative care.

All of the interviewees were contacted first by telephone and asked if they would consent to an interview of one to one and a half hours. Anonymity was assured. Interviews took place in the alternative practice setting, in hospitals or in the interviewee's home. The interviews were semi-structured and covered a wide array of topics relating to the individual's background and training, motivations, experience in practice, and modes of negotiating among different health practice cultures. The interviews were conducted by two graduate students in the Department of Sociology and Anthropology of the Hebrew University of Jerusalem in 2004–5 under the supervision of the senior author.[1] All interviews were taped with the agreement of the interviewees and were subsequently transcribed into systematic computerised records. These texts provided the raw material for the substantive analysis. Intensive reading and re-reading of the texts led to the identification of the principal themes which concerned boundary work as rhetorical devices and to related practices utilised in the work context (Adams 2004; Allen 2000; Gieryn 1999). Written sources and documents relating to the practice of nursing and midwifery in Israel and elsewhere served to contextualise the data from the interviews.

Findings

The findings will be presented in three sections: 'structural characteristics and their implications'; 'values and norms'; and 'role performance: some significant others'. In each section the material will be presented separately for nurses and midwives while intra-professional patterns will be noted in each group. Finally, a comparative analysis will highlight the principal differences between the two groups.

Structural characteristics and their implications

Nurses

The nurses who engage in alternative health care are characterised by multiplicity with regard to the settings and content of their work. Most were employed full time or part time in a biomedical institution as conventional nurses and worked after hours in a private clinic providing alternative health care. Such clinics were located in their home or adjacent to it. A small number of older or retired interviewees had relinquished conventional nursing and practised only alternative health care in their own private clinics.

Multiplicity is also seen in the numerous fields of alternative health care engaged in by individual nurses. One versatile practitioner reported that she had trained and now worked in homeopathy, Feldenkreis, reflexology, reiki, Bach flowers and biofeedback – utilising one or more of these specialisations in accordance with the patient's needs. In the privacy of their alternative clinics, nurses are autonomous in their practice. They evoke biomedical practices to establish credibility and legitimacy with clients; but the heart of their practice is their alternative knowledge and the alternative techniques which they use.

In the course of their work in the context of biomedical institutions, a more cautious, conservative approach is taken. Even when they have doubts about some of the hospital practices or are critical of physicians' attitudes, the nurses know that overt deviance could cost them their reputation or even their job; conformity to biomedical norms, especially in a public context, is viewed as the safest form of behaviour:

> I am an employee of the hospital and must keep to its rules . . . I don't want any trouble.

The nurses are aware that the boundaries of biomedical organisations are strongly guarded and, for the most part, the guardians do not welcome alternative health ideas and practices. Biomedical reference groups are recognised as powerful and potentially censorious; they could threaten a nurse's credibility – or delegitimise her by defining her as 'far out'. Most nurses are reluctant to let their biomedical colleagues and supervisors know of their alternative practice:

> I never speak of my other [CAM] clinic when I'm in the hospital . . . why should I look for trouble with the head of the department?

Nevertheless, several of the nurses interviewed are convinced of the desirability of importing alternative methods into hospitals and clinics because of their conviction that they improve patient care. Some of the more enterprising are willing to undertake this risk – but are careful to ensure two conditions: the patient's consent; and assurance that they are not observed by other biomedical personnel:

> I always ask the patient first . . . and look around to make sure no other nurses or doctors can see what I'm doing.

Midwives

All of the midwives interviewed in this study worked routinely in delivery rooms of public hospitals, full time or part time. A small number also offer pre-natal care within the context of the hospital programme or privately. Thus most of the alternative care provided by midwives is given within the context of a biomedical hospital. All uncomplicated births are delivered by licensed midwives in hospitals, i.e. 80 per cent of all births. The midwives and their support personnel constitute the active staff of the delivery rooms; physicians are generally situated in adjacent locations and are summoned by the midwife only in case of need. This structural differentiation unambiguously defines the physician's domain as one of 'pathology' while the midwife's territory is formally limited to 'uncomplicated' births (i.e. healthy, non-problematic births).

The alternative fields of practice used by midwives include a variety of therapies which focus on techniques used during labour and childbirth although some relate to pre-natal and post-natal care. Reflecting the emphasis of the preparatory course (referred to above), the interviews indicate that the most frequently utilised techniques applied by the midwives were reflexology, reiki, imaging and massage techniques to promote natural childbirth. In the relative freedom of their practice setting, midwives are able to exercise initiatives in introducing CAM to predisposed consumers. Their confidence in doing this is bolstered by the 'virtual' presence of physicians – who are on call in case of need. At the same time the midwives relish their autonomy which is fully legitimised by the medical community. In a new birthing facility at an elite hospital in the Tel Aviv area, one midwife stated proudly,

> there are no doctors around . . . we midwives run everything . . . it's a wonderful feeling.

Upon arrival in the delivery room, a woman in labour is assigned to an attending midwife. It is difficult to estimate the proportion of midwives using CAM but those interested in utilising alternative methods see every arrival as a potential client. They are careful to obtain informed consent and to respond to requests for conventional procedures during labour – if the woman is unwilling to continue with alternative techniques. It is axiomatic that life-threatening conditions call for biomedical intervention. But some midwives exercise their independence and even venture to challenge the physician's stance:

> when the doctor said that I should give her epidural to speed things up, I spoke to the woman to see if she was willing to wait a bit longer . . . and then I said to the doctor, 'let's wait for a bit'; he said, 'OK, but only for two more hours' and I replied quietly, 'perhaps we can wait till morning' (five more hours) and the doctor agreed with me.

Values and norms

Nurses

The nurses interviewed expressed a wide variety of beliefs and norms concerning CAM. The heterogeneity of their views reflects variation in their formal training, the nature of their workplace, and the large number of areas of alternative practice in which they engage. While they have in common their basic training as qualified nurses, they vary in terms of supplementary biomedical training: a few qualified as surgical, paediatric or public health nurses while some did not continue their training in nursing specialties. Their training and practice in alternative care range over a wide range of the alternative options; furthermore they deal with a great variety of health problems. This structural heterogeneity yielded considerable variation in the nurses' position on the values and norms that guide their alternative practice. The themes discussed below – while not common to all – were widely expressed by the nurses interviewed.

CONFIDENCE IN BIOMEDICINE

The specialised knowledge of the physician establishes a boundary of authority. This is accepted and respected by nurses and there is no evidence for a desire to cross this line. They carefully avoid expressing any criticism in the presence of patients. Life-threatening conditions provide an absolute marker for the priority of biomedical intervention. Several nurses referred to the formal responsibility of doctors and to the potential dangers of legal action if they are not consulted for serious, life-threatening medical conditions. This stance reflects a tradition of respect for the physician's authority and knowledge but is also a self-protecting mechanism to avoid legal complications in their own practice.

I ask the patient if she/he has been to see a doctor. If they say, 'No, I preferred to see you', I say, 'I am not a doctor; first you must see a doctor for tests . . . then I'll decide on your treatment.'

Many nurses accept the research standards and methodology advocated by biomedical professionals. Most take blood pressure, pulse, measure height and weight; almost all request results of blood tests, X-rays, computerised tomographic (CT) examinations and other relevant information obtained in the course of biomedical care.

NURSING AS A SOURCE OF PRIDE AND CONFIDENCE

Some alternative nurses are overtly proud of their biomedical origin and training believing it enhances their ability to diagnose a problem and provide high quality alternative care:

It's because I'm a trained nurse that I know when to send a patient to the doctor . . . my background in nursing helps me all the time.

CRITICISM OF BIOMEDICINE

Several nurses were overtly critical of physicians especially with regard to their over-reliance on technology and medication, invasive practices, separation of mind and body and inadequate sensitivity to the needs of patients:

What bothers me about doctors is their insensitivity to patients' needs, their cold, impersonal attitude and lack of real human contact with sick persons . . . their dependence of machine and tests.

Several nurses emphasised their holistic approach to health care: the integral relationship of body and mind. They tend to emphasise the latter, constructing their role as providers of support, empathy and compassion. Since these are not provided by physicians who concentrate exclusively on the body, the alternative nurses perceive themselves as 'specialists' in providing integrated care:

doctors never have time to really get to know a patient . . . they're always rushed . . . I make it a point to let the patient feel that I am there to listen, to feel the problem along with her.

PATIENT AUTONOMY

Nurses in alternative practice support patient autonomy and encourage the women in their care to assert their independence *vis-à-vis* their biomedical practitioner.

> I say to patients 'you should depend on yourself and on your own good judgement, if you feel the level of your sugar is improving, go to your doctor and tell him so . . . ask him to reduce the level of your medication.'

INCORPORATING ALTERNATIVE CARE INTO MAINSTREAM BIOMEDICINE

As noted, most nurses who have adopted alternative methods remain inherently loyal to biomedicine and are not troubled by epistemological differences. Several were adamant in denying any conflict or competition between biomedicine and CAM. They view their alternative care as an expansion of biomedical care by means of additional techniques. They are convinced that they can help patients in areas in which biomedicine has been unable to provide effective care through the use of safe, effective methods.

Many of these nurses prefer the term 'complementary' to 'alternative'. This provides a rhetorical device which expresses their recognition of the centrality of biomedicine and their construction of their own role as supportive of that position – a rhetorical presentation also identified from the analysis of general practitioners' (GPs') accounts of their CAM practice (Adams 2004). In effect, the nurses see no reason why they should not be recognised and incorporated into mainstream biomedicine as additional specialists who are skilled in providing a much needed element of care.

> Our work is not an alternative to medicine. We are complementary . . . that is to say that we add other methods . . . there is no conflict only more methods to reduce patients' suffering.

Midwives

In terms of their training and practice skills – biomedical and alternative – the midwives interviewed are a more homogeneous group than the nurses. This differential homogeneity is based on a structural difference between the groups: the midwives' professional work focuses on a 'single issue': childbirth, while the nurses provide care for a wide range of health problems. The midwives are more homogeneous in terms of their formal biomedical training: all are qualified nurses with one specialty (i.e. midwifery). Although they have been trained and practise a variety of alternative practices, all of these relate to one area: child birth. This may help explain the fact that our analysis showed more consensus among the midwives who were also more explicit in stating their underlying beliefs than the nurses. While individual nurses mentioned some of the beliefs noted below, they were divided in their views. It will be noted that there is considerable overlap in the norms and values of the two groups.

CONFIDENCE IN BIOMEDICINE

Working primarily within the framework of biomedical institutions, the midwives express their respect and admiration for medical knowledge and achievements. They view their alternative practices as additional tools and techniques within a biomedical framework. In this regard the midwives view their alternative practice as an expansion of the boundaries of the biomedical system:

> the medical profession does wonderful things . . . saves lives . . . we are not doctors but we help and add a lot of extra techniques that reduce suffering and pain. I believe we should be part of the overall medical care system.

CRITICAL STANCE TOWARDS OVER-USE OF 'TECHNOLOGY'

Midwives are virtually unanimous in their overt objection, sometimes expressed in heated tones, to the over-use of technology and to its negative effects. They are critical of physicians who emphasise rationalised, routinised tests and technically prescribed procedures:

> monitoring the baby's progress has turned into a search for pathologies which in most cases are not there or go away by themselves.

> it makes no sense to assume that every birth is a high risk; every woman does not need to be on the monitor – 85 per cent of births are completely normal and need no medical intervention.

> Epidural is the opium of hospitals . . . it is used as a 'silencer' to keep things quiet, unemotional and under control.

Part of the objection to an overly technical orientation stems from a belief in holism: the individual is viewed as an inseparable whole in which physical and emotional needs are intimately related:

> there is a unity of mind and body; the body is not a machine.

EMPHASIS ON NATURAL PROCESSES

The belief in natural childbirth is a dominant theme that is common to all of the midwives interviewed and is a central tenet of their alternative practice.

> Giving birth is a healthy phenomenon, part of the natural flow of life. Interference in this normal process which is common to all living creatures can only have negative effects.

Pain in giving birth is considered by these midwives to be natural but is not 'good' or desirable in itself. They suggest it can be eased considerably by a variety of alternative methods so as to allow the natural processes to progress at their own pace and that an epidural should be used only if the woman feels that the pain is unbearable:

> let nature take its own time. I object to speeding up labour; it's better not to use epidural to reduce pain but rather massage and other techniques that are not invasive or drug-based.

INTUITION, FEELING, EMOTION

The indeterminate 'I' component of care plays a central role in the professional orientation of midwives engaged in alternative practice. As used by Jamous and Pelouille (1970) the 'I' component refers to knowledge that is not entirely rational, is partly intuitive and is located in the domain of individual interpretation and judgement. Midwives in alternative practice emphasise the centrality of 'I' by referring to women's feelings, emotions and need for support during childbirth – frequently highlighting the uniqueness, meaningfulness and spirituality of the context in which they work:

> as soon as I meet a woman when she arrives at the delivery room, I can feel – just by looking at her – whether she will consent to have alternative treatment . . . it's my intuition and I've never been wrong.

> every birth is different, individual . . . it's never the same . . . and its success depends on the intuition of the woman and of the midwife . . . you can't do it 'by the book'.

EMPOWERMENT OF WOMEN

Many alternative midwives adhere to a type of feminism that focuses on the empowerment of women through the experience of childbirth. A natural birth is viewed as a great accomplishment and serves to give women a sense of achievement and power:

the midwife looked deep into the eyes of the woman and said triumphantly, 'you did it!' in order to give her a sense of triumph, of having done a splendid and wonderful thing.

NOSTALGIA

Many midwives express a nostalgic longing for a past which is viewed as simpler, more 'authentic' and less encumbered by technologies. It is viewed as better than the present and imbued with greater 'truth'. This stance parallels Tovey and Adams' (2003) view that the current interest in alternative methods can be viewed as a continuation or revival of earlier patterns which focus more on emotional needs and patient-centred practice. As one midwife explains:

> in ancient Egypt we know that midwives used touch methods to help against pain . . . and even now we are told by immigrant women who came here from Morocco that they gave birth with midwives who helped them with massage and herbal brews.

Some midwives express a longing for the earlier role of the midwife – when she performed a variety of tasks which added up to a meaningful whole. In those days her expertise included knowledge and use of herbal products, massage techniques, positioning the woman for comfort and ease during labour, delivering the baby, provision of support and help after birth in breast feeding and infant care. In recent years, task differentiation has transferred many of her traditional tasks to other specialists, leaving her with an emasculated role:

> delivery of twins and shifting the position of the baby in the womb are done by doctors because they are seen as risky. Yoga teachers and others have taken over the preparatory tasks, baby nurses take over the care of the child immediately after birth, specialists in breast feeding and care of newborn infants offer post-partum help – all we midwives can do is deliver normal births.

Contemporary methods of delivery and infant care are thought to be accompanied by numerous pathological effects which were rarely seen in the past: allergies to non-breast milk, digestive problems, breast infections, temperature after birth, loss of the bonding experience of breast feeding and the ill-effects of drugs.

A MISSION

Many of the alternative midwives feel that they have a mission, a 'calling' to spread the message regarding the important contribution of their approach in improving the birthing experience: reducing fear, increasing a sense of achievement, and strengthening the relationship with the child. This orientation is often accompanied by considerable zeal and passion:

> this may sound presumptuous, but I feel I have an important mission, it's like a religious feeling, this is not only a job – I have a 'vocation' in my life to let people know that there are alternatives available.

In their enthusiasm and commitment, some of the midwives criticised their colleagues who were less imbued with a sense of mission, referring to them as 'bureaucratic' in their approach:

> many midwives have no real emotional commitment to their work, they don't feel the experience of each woman as a meaningful one . . . it's like a mass-production line.

Role performance: some significant others

Nurses

Some of the alternative nurses view conventional nursing as a dreary, unstimulating, dead-end occupation. They perceive their hospital work as technical and routine, geared to support the work of the physicians. A number expressed resentment toward the doctors who are unwilling to allow an expansion of the nurse's role to include more curative work:

> what does a nurse do besides wash patients, take their temperature? The doctors won't let them do anything else. Nurses never do anything really important to help patients.

Nurses tend to distinguish between the medical profession as a whole which is generally perceived as derisive of alternative methods – and selected professionals who are supportive. Thus one nurse whose private clinic was in a kibbutz stated:

> After many years of working alongside Dr M. we have a real understanding and he refers many patients to me.

But another felt a total lack of communication:

> We speak different languages . . . I feel I'm speaking Chinese and he is speaking Hottentot language.

Several nurses stated that in recent years physicians are more tolerant and accepting of selected alternative practices than they were in the past:

> In the past doctors were all against our methods . . . but in recent years they are more and more accepting.

Midwives

As noted, midwives are careful to obtain a woman's consent before initiating CAM treatment. Having obtained this and continuing to check for 'complications' in the course of labour or birth, the midwives are confident in utilising CAM practices. Their confidence is bolstered by the many obstetricians who support natural childbirth whenever it is possible. A general commitment to 'natural' childbirth provides a shared ideological approach across the cognitive boundary of biomedicine and CAM; it encompasses many obstetricians and midwives who do not practise CAM. While other differences inevitably remain to separate CAM and biomedical practitioners, this is one of the important areas that eases boundary crossing.

Like the nurses, many midwives expressed the optimistic view that physicians are coming to accept CAM increasingly in recent years. An interesting presence in the delivery room are 'doulas': non-professional women who assist women during childbirth (Kennell et al. 1991; Langer et al. 1998; Martin et al. 1998; McGrath and Kennell 1998). The work of the doula includes the non-clinical aspects of care during childbirth, i.e. emotional reassurance, warmth, comfort, encouragement and respect. She offers help and advice on measures such as breathing, relaxation, movement and positioning; doulas do not perform clinical tasks, such as vaginal exams or foetal heart rate monitoring. In Israel, doulas are hired by some women preparing for birth, to accompany them to the delivery room and remain throughout the labour and birthing process as well as their aftermath.

The daily pressures of work in the delivery room are described by midwives as extremely demanding so that in many cases they are less able than the doula to focus on the emotional needs of individual women; they feel that these pressures push them into the routine, technical aspects of care while the doula, who is there for only one woman, is able to devote her full time to providing her with support. There is an undercurrent of resentment among the midwives caused by the 'usurpation' by the doulas of their core supportive role. In fact much of the midwives' work routine involves 'technical' tasks: attachment and supervision of foetal monitoring, the rupture of the membrane, attachment and monitoring IV fluid intake.

> The doula is there for one woman . . . I have to deal with many . . . so I don't have time to give her all my attention to one . . . The doulas have taken over an important part of our job.

> sometimes I'm jealous of the doulas because they do what I want to do.

But other midwives try to perform in all areas, despite the pressure.

> Yes, I'm very busy . . . but if I really try, I can find the time to sit with her while she's having contractions . . . give her some reflexological treatment . . . a bit of aromatherapy . . . in between doing everything else.

Others – in the spirit of professional role differentiation – feel that midwives and doulas work well together – complementing each other's roles. It is paradoxical that in the relationship of the two in the delivery room context, a reversal takes place: the midwife comes to represent the technical element of care while the doula specialises in emotional support. This structure is reinforced by the fact that the midwife – and not the doula – is in direct contact with the physician via the monitor and other biomedical procedures.

> while she [the doula] holds the patient's hand and comforts her, I devote myself to the more technical parts of birthing.

Even when the doula is present in the delivery room, she is not part of the system. Her outsider status makes it possible for her to 'represent' the woman *vis-à-vis* the hospital staff and even to criticise the physician – an act which most midwives, who are regular members of the hospital staff, are reluctant to undertake:

> the doula is the only one who dares to ask the doctors 'embarrassing' questions . . . she is not afraid of them because she is not part of the system.

Discussion – comparative analysis

We will first focus on themes common to nurses and midwives who engage in alternative practice and then highlight differences between them. Intra-professional patterns will be pointed out.

Common characteristics

Both groups assert their loyalty to and confidence in biomedicine and re-assert their desire to remain within its cognitive and epistemological boundaries. This is seen in expressions of admiration for the achievements of medicine and its life-saving accomplishments. Both groups make clear their reliance on and use of biomedical tests and treatment methods. Nurses and midwives – however committed they are to alternative methods – make clear the cognitive and practice boundary beyond which they will not venture: this is defined as the exclusive domain of biomedicine. High risk, danger to life, need for specialised medical skills or knowledge – all signal immediate relegation of responsibility to a physician and postponement or withdrawal of alternative care.

Neither group challenges the epistemological boundaries of biomedicine but both are critical of its practice modes and seek to expand the boundaries of bio-practice to include alternative methods. In both groups the view is frequently expressed that CAM does not represent an 'alternative' or a challenge to biomedicine; it should be viewed as an extension of the practice techniques of biomedicine and be legitimately included in its domain. This view is bolstered rhetorically by use of the term 'complementary' and avoidance of the concept 'alternative'.

Both nurses and midwives are unstinting in the criticism they address to the modes of practice and orientation of many physicians. This disapproval focuses on two substantive issues both of which refer to the epistemological issues of mind and body, also referred to as 'holism': (a) over-use of technology and drugs; and (b) failure to take account of patients' feelings and emotions or to extend support and empathy. Both groups see themselves as specialists in b. Because of the centrality of their belief in natural childbirth, the midwives show a fervent concern with a.

Both groups express optimism with regard to the increase over time in the acceptance of alternative methods by doctors. While many physicians continue to reject and even to denigrate the research that has been done to evaluate alternative methods, there is evidence of collusion by increasing numbers of physicians who refer patients to CAM practitioners and who accept specific alternative methods even when they are unable to place them analytically in the context of biomedical thinking. These utilise an instrumental criterion for legitimation, i.e. the 'proof of the pudding' phenomenon, expressed in clinical effectiveness. This is seen in the oft-mentioned remark by doctors, 'I don't know why it works, but it does work'.

Both groups are client-dependent in their need to obtain the patient's consent to accept CAM. And both face major reservations – if not hostility – from numerous other biomedical practitioners. Many in both groups are active sponsors of CAM in an attempt to gain more legitimation.

Differences

Structural heterogeneity among the nurses results in considerable intra-professional variation in the norms and values expressed. This is not the case with the midwives. Structural homogeneity in their formal training, along with a focus on the specific area of childbirth, result in considerable homogeneity among the midwives with regard to the values and norms which define their professional behaviour. This may be viewed as their 'epistemology' – although it is not formally labelled as such. We use the term to refer to a set of core axioms mentioned by almost all the midwives resulting in little intra-professional variation among them in this area.

The midwives' 'epistemology' includes the common values noted above – confidence in biomedicine along with criticism of physicians' over-reliance on technology and drugs as well as their insensitivity to patients' feelings and emotional needs, optimism as to growing acceptance of CAM by selected physicians – but also consensual views on the following values: an emphasis on natural processes, empowerment of women through childbirth, nostalgia for the past when childbirth was a more meaningful experience and midwifery was a more broadly defined occupation, a sense of mission to spread their message. While a few nurses also referred to the latter values, others did not refer to them at all during the interviews.

These common beliefs provide the midwives with a stronger sense of cohesive solidarity than is evident among the nurses. Since, like nurses and physicians, they also adhere to the basic tenets of biomedical epistemology – it may be said that they are characterised by a more broadly contoured set of values and beliefs than either of the other groups. The boundaries of their common epistemology extend beyond those defined by biomedicine.

A difference noted between the two groups is seen in the quality of their commitment to CAM. Among the midwives, we noted more of a zealous commitment, a sense of mission, a 'calling' to spread the word on these methods accompanied by a fervent belief in their importance and efficacy. For a few, their work in alternative health care was part of a larger, multi-faceted complex of 'new-age' beliefs and behaviour.

A major structural difference distinguishes the two groups in their efforts to introduce CAM into biomedical contexts. Again this difference is associated with the extent of insulation of the locus of their alternative practice and in the general orientation of their principal professional reference groups.

The nurses locate most of their CAM practice in settings separated spatially from their biomedical setting of practice: generally in a private clinic where they are completely independent and confident. Thus an unambiguous geographical boundary separates their biomedical and CAM practice.

At the same time, most of the nurses also work in biomedical institutions where the boundaries of biomedical legitimacy are unambiguously drawn. An interesting intra-professional difference is seen between the more and the less confident and enterprising among them. For the most part nurses prefer to play by the rules of the game in biomedical contexts, i.e. keeping their alternative practices out of view. At the same time, the more dedicated among them seek to introduce selected alternative techniques into hospitals or clinics despite the risks such efforts may pose: censure, being labelled as 'far out' or even sacked. Therefore these efforts are carried out with extreme caution and are generally clandestine.

The midwives, on the other hand, are employed in delivery rooms of biomedical hospitals where they enjoy considerable autonomy. As long as labour and delivery are deemed 'uncomplicated', the midwives are in complete charge. For the most part, the physician's presence is virtual, i.e. maintained through the monitor. Once they have obtained the woman's consent, they feel free to introduce alternative techniques to control labour pains and reduce use of drugs. Their self-confidence is bolstered by the knowledge that many of the obstetricians support the ideal of natural childbirth.

Under these conditions they are relatively free to use CAM in the delivery room thus expanding the boundary of CAM legitimacy into the heartland of biomedicine. These structural differences are relevant to the nurses' and midwives' dependence on the physician's authority in drawing the boundary of legitimacy with regard to their practice of CAM. With respect to the midwives: the physician's presence – virtual or real – in the delivery room provides an unambiguous message indicating when CAM treatment must be terminated, i.e. when the birth is 'complicated'. Thus the midwives' use of CAM is contingent on the pathology of the case as defined by biomedical criteria. In the case of CAM nurses: their patients can opt to use both bio medical treatment and CAM – more or less simultaneously, i.e. if they are ambulatory, they do not need to give up one in favour of the other. In deciding when CAM is inappropriate, the nurses make that decision on their own – basing it on their own knowledge and training in biomedicine.

The presence of doulas in the delivery rooms highlights another of the boundary dilemmas faced by midwives. The doulas specialise in the provision of emotional reassurance, warmth, comfort and encouragement during labour, birth and its aftermath. These skills focus directly on one of the essential elements of the midwives' professional role; what is more, the doula, working exclusively with one woman, can deliver these qualities unstintingly while midwives are under pressure to care for the urgent needs of several women simultaneously.

In a sense, the doula makes it possible for the midwife to move to a more differentiated professional level by leaving the less demanding, lesser skilled tasks to a less-trained person. This is not appreciated by those midwives who feel that the emotional component is central to their work. There is pressure in the delivery room for the midwives to work in the technically orientated enclave of biomedicine while the doula 'takes over' the affective heart of CAM midwifery. This situation creates an additional intra-professional cleavage between those alternative midwives who resent the doula and those who feel she plays a positive supportive role.

In sum, the outcome of these patterns is that midwives and nurses prac-tising CAM share an important set of norms and values. At the same time, the midwives are a more cohesive group who adhere on a consensual basis to an additional set of values and salient experiences which are anchored in their unique position as legitimate insiders in the biomedical establish-ment. While nurses report occasional, clandestine introduction of CAM in their hospital practice, most of their CAM practice takes place in the security of settings which are spatially isolated from biomedical institutions.

The midwives engage in CAM with greater confidence and transparency inside biomedical settings. This means that they have successfully crossed the organisational boundary of biomedicine and practise comfortably within it. Their self-assurance is reinforced by the full responsibility they carry for 80 per cent of the births (which are 'uncomplicated'). The findings show that there is some flexibility in the definition of 'uncomplicated' and determined CAM midwives sometimes negotiate the boundaries of that condition. Finally, the fact that many obstetricians support the notion of 'natural' childbirth provides them with legitimation for many of their CAM practices.

Note

1 The senior author would like to thank Liat Lifschitz who interviewed the nurses and Sky Gross who interviewed the midwives.

References

Adams, J. (2004) Demarcating the medical/non-medical border: occupational boundary-work within GPs' accounts of their integrative practice. In Tovey, P., Easthope, G. and Adams, J. (eds) *The Mainstreaming of Complementary and Alternative Medicine: Studies in Social Context*. London: Routledge, pp. 140–57.

Allen, D. (2000) Doing occupational demarcation: the boundary-work of nurse managers in a district hospital. *Journal of Contemporary Ethnography* 29(3): 326–56.

Bergman, R. (1986) Academisation of nursing education: the Israeli experience. *Journal of Advanced Nursing* 11: 225–9.

Coburn, D. and Willis, E. (2000) The medical profession: knowledge, power and autonomy. In Albrecht, G. L., Fitzpatrick, R. and Scrimshaw, S. (eds) *Handbook of Social Studies in Health and Medicine*. Thousand Oaks, CA: Sage, pp. 377–93.

Gieryn, T. F. (1999) *Cultural Boundaries of Science: Credibility on the Line*. Chicago, IL: University of Chicago Press.

Glazer, S. (2000) Therapeutic touch and postmodern nursing. *Knowledge and Society* 12: 319–41.

Hirschkorn, K. A. and Bourgeault, I. L. (2005) Conceptualizing mainstream health care providers' behaviours in relation to complementary and alternative medicine. *Social Science & Medicine* 61(1): 157–70.

Hoffmann, F. L. (1991) Feminism and nursing. *The National Woman Studies Association Journal* 3(1): 53–69.

Hojat, M. et al. (2003) Comparisons of American, Israeli, Italian and Mexican physicians and nurses on the total and factor scores of the Jefferson scale of attitudes toward physician–nurse collaborative relationships. *International Journal of Nursing Studies* 40(4): 427–35.

Jamous, H. and Pelouille, B. (1970) Changes in the French university-hospital system. In Jackson, J. A. (ed.) *Professions and Professionalisation.* Cambridge: Cambridge University Press, pp. 111–52.

Johnson, M. B. (1990) The holistic paradigm in nursing: the diffusion of an innovation. *Research in Nursing and Health* 13: 129–39.

Kennell, J. H., Klaus, M. H., McGrath, S. K., Robertson, S. and Hinkley, C. (1991) Continuous emotional support during labour in a US hospital: a randomised controlled trial. *JAMA* 265: 2197–201.

Langer, A., Campero, L., Garcia, C. and Reynoso, S. (1998) Effects of psychosocial support during labour and childbirth on breast feeding, medical interventions, and mothers' well-being in a Mexican public hospital: a randomised clinical trial. *British Journal of Obstetrics and Gynaecology* 105: 1056–63.

Martin, S., Landry, S., Steelman, L., Kennell, J. H. and McGrath, S. (1998) The effect of doula support during labour on mother–infant interaction at 2 months. *Infant Behavior Development* 21: 556.

McGrath, S. K. and Kennell, J. H. (1998) Induction of labour and doula support. *Pediatric Res.* 43(4): Part II, 14A.12.

Mizrachi, N. and Shuval, J. T. (2005) Beween formal and enacted policy: changing the contours of boundaries. *Social Science & Medicine* 60(7): 1611–60.

Mizrachi, N., Shuval, J. T. and Gross, S. (2005) Boundary at work: alternative medicine in biomedical settings. *Sociology of Health and Illness* 27(1): 20–43.

Reches, R. (1978) Midwifery in Israel: tradition and progress. In Reches, R. (ed.) Midwifery in Israel: on the services provided to women in Israel. Paper for the International Congress of Midwifery, 1978. Hebrew. Unpublished.

Salvage, J. (1992) The new nursing: empowering patients or empowering nurses? In Robinson, J., Gray, A. and Elkan R. (eds) *Policy Issues in Nursing.* Milton Keynes: Open University Press, pp. 9–23.

Shmueli, A. and Shuval, J. (2003) Consultations with non-conventional medicine providers: 2000 vs. 1993. *Israel Medical Association Journal* 6, January: 3–8.

Shmueli, A. and Shuval, J. (2006) Satisfaction with family physicians and specialists and the use of CAM in Israel. *Evidence-based Complementary and Alternative Medicine* 3(2): 273–8.

Shuval, J. T. and Anson, O. (2000) *Ha'Ikar Habriut: Social Structure and Health in Israel.* Jerusalem: Magnes Press. (In Hebrew.)

Shuval, J. T. (2001) Collaborative relationships of alternative practitioners and physicians in Israel: an exploratory study. *Complementary Health Practice Review* 7(2): 111–25.

Shuval, J. T., Mizrachi, N. and Smetannikov, E. (2002) Entering the well-guarded fortress: alternative practitioners in hospital settings. *Social Science & Medicine* 55(10): 1745–55.

Shuval, J. T. and Mizrachi, N. (2004) Changing boundaries: modes of co-existence of alternative and biomedicine. *Qualitative Health Research* 14(5): 675–90.

Tel-Oren, A. (2000) Home births in Israel. Israel Midwives Association: http://www.midwives.co.il (In Hebrew.)

Tovey, P. and Adams, J. (2003) Nostalgic and nostophobic referencing and the authentication of nurses' use of complementary therapies. *Social Science & Medicine* 56(7): 1469–80.

Zwanger, L. (1988) The historical process of the academization of nursing education in Israel. In *Proceedings of the 11th Annual Meeting of the Workgroup of European Nurse-Researchers, Jerusalem.* New York: Oxford University Press, pp. 10–28.

Part III

Public health and patient issues

Chapter 7

'Latent' and 'realised' risk cultures

Woman-centred midwifery and CAM

Karen Lane

Introduction: risk assessment and midwifery

Beck's (1992) concept of the Risk Society encapsulates a tectonic shift from a focus on class consciousness of the 'first modernity' to risk consciousness and individualisation of 'the second modernity'. Specifically, the goal to eliminate scarcity under class society is substituted for the eradication of fear and risk caused by technological change under the risk society (Scott 2002). Within the health arena, medicalisation (a focus on illness and disease) is supplanted by biomedicalisation (a focus on health and risk). Health becomes an individual life project or achievement rather than a static physical state where the role of health professionals is to assist individuals to avoid and control *potential* risks, typically through technological surveillance (Clark et al. 2003). Within maternity care, for example, obstetricians and midwives base their professionalism on the successful anticipation of risk before it occurs. The contentious point is that these professions employ different models of birth and the body in their understanding of the sites of risk and its avoidance. The techno-rational/scientific (biomedical) model has assumed that the body itself is inherently risky. The role of the obstetrician, therefore, is to anticipate risk before it occurs typically intervening to avoid an adverse outcome. In reverse order, holistic midwifery regards medical interventions as the major source of risk to women and babies (Lane 1995) because for midwives, birth is a normal physiological and social event (Skinner 2006: 62); midwives avoid risk by avoiding medical intervention – that is, in facilitating a normal birth through 'woman-centred' care. Consumerism has thus traditionally formed the corner-stone of midwifery practice and professionalisation. However, while cognisant of the relationship between risk assessment and woman-centred care and the wider project of midwifery professionalisation, this chapter focuses primarily upon a critical examination of the rise of consumerism and risk cultures and how they relate to the growing support for complementary and alternative medicine (CAM) within midwifery.

In this chapter I argue that 'woman-centred care' within midwifery practices is inherently compatible with CAM and focus attention upon two advantages that CAM provides midwifery. First, as a signifier of the individualisation of health care with its more recent shift towards consumerism, CAM facilitates the active participation of consumers in making decisions about their own health care. Just as CAM recognises individual idiosyncrasies in proposing appropriate treatment, so is midwifery cognisant of the active participation of the mother in defining her own care compatible with her unique biography. CAM may profitably add to the midwifery arsenal of treatment regimes in which case it would help to define midwifery as a 'realised' risk culture.

The second advantage for midwives using CAM is that it allows midwives to practise as primary carers effectively and autonomously in managing real and perceived risk without recourse to medical expertise. CAM promotes midwifery as primary care (rather than obstetric assistance) because CAM lies outside of the medical jurisdiction and thus facilitates midwives' professional distance from their institutional competitors and colonisers (i.e. obstetrics). Midwifery and CAM are thus natural allies but only if CAM is adopted as part of a 'transformative integration' pattern of medicine (one that refuses to compromise holistic principles and is used only in consultation with the woman) (Kailin 2001; Coulter 2004).

Risk Society thesis: the heartland of health care, obstetrics, midwifery and childbirth

At the heart of the Risk Society thesis (Beck et al. 1994; Adam and van Loon 2002) is the proposition that modern societies are the structured outcome of advanced industrialisation, a process that has produced hazards that cannot be controlled or managed by existing safety systems. Our faith in the progressive nature of science is a casualty of the new risk society because science, in conjunction with commercial exploitation, has been a key actor in producing the very risks it now seeks to resolve. The revelation of the fallibility of science produces the first proposition of the risk society – 'reflexive modernisation' which refers to the self-authorisation of individuals as a consequence of their mass disenchantment of science. Individual autonomy is the outcome of negotiating contradictory discourses emanating from scientific inquiry and in finding their own resolutions for scientific and commercially produced hazards. The second proposition is that the risks manufactured by industrial technologies are dispersed globally, unevenly and often invisibly; they materialise only as symptoms perhaps some time later.

A more recent update entails a further proposition that risks are manufactured by social individuals from particular vantage points or philosophical traditions. Risks are not simply 'out there' but based upon context, epistemology, political interest and power; risks are attached to situated knowledge (Haraway 1988). It follows that there are competing definitions of risk associated with competing paradigms of knowledge that produce competing solutions and, since this is a political process, not all definitions and their respective solutions will be equally credible. The political process centrally involves the media, commerce, the state, law and science – all of whom produce variable interpretations of the meaning of risks. The outcome is a pervasive sense of uncertainty apprehended by reflexive individuals in different ways that call for a reflexive disciplinarity; an opening up of knowledge claims that go beyond traditional disciplinary boundaries. This is what is inferred by 'reflexive modernisation' (Beck 1992) and what Adam and van Loon (2002: 10–11) call a 'repositioning of risk' requiring a 'repositioning' of the bases of social theory. The latter must necessarily relinquish an ambition to produce theory that will provide general laws and abstractions as in the Enlightenment quest for prediction and order, or determinate judgement, in favour of theory that harnesses what Lash (2002) calls 'an aesthetic of the sublime'; a judgement based upon bodily powers of tacticity, the immediate and the sensuous.

Similarly, Scott (2002: 38) argues, Beck's theory of the risk society anticipates risks as really 'out there'; it is an objectivist, realist theory of risk. Scott denies an unmediated connection between risk consciousness and real risks on the grounds that this ignores the interpretation of risk by different kinds of communities with their specific conventions, norms and structures. Scott is reluctant to concede Beck's division between the class consciousness of class societies and the risk consciousness of risk society, an argument that rests on the indivisibility between risk consciousness and class consciousness. It assumes that those who have most to lose are those who perceive higher levels of risk. The question for Scott (2002: 43) is, 'how safe is safe enough for this particular culture?' – to answer this question we must inquire into the relative and dynamic nature of the discourses surrounding individual freedoms and collective responsibility within a particular society.

Risk Culture

In adopting a social constructivist paradigm, 'Risk Culture' is the starting point for Lash (2002: 47) who, like Douglas and Wildavsky (1983), argues that 'real' risks have not necessarily increased but that our perceptions of risk have escalated. Beck et al.'s (1994) objectivist notion of risk *society* assumes 'a determinate, institutional, normative, rule bound and necessarily hierarchical ordering of individual members in regard to their utilitarian interests' whereas:

> Risk *cultures*, by contrast, presume not a determinate ordering, but a reflexive or indeterminate disordering . . . Their media are not procedural

norms but substantive values. Their governing figurations are not rules but symbols: they are less a hierarchical ordering than a horizontal disordering. Their fluid quasi-membership is as likely to be collective as individual, and their concern is less with utilitarian interests than the fostering of the good life . . . Risk cultures are based less in cognitive than in aesthetic reflexivity. Risk cultures are reflexive communities.

(Lash 2002: 47; emphasis added)

To substantiate his departure from a positivist view of risk, Lash draws critically upon Douglas and Wildavsky's thesis in *Risk and Culture* (1983) proposing there are no increases in risk but only an increase in the perception of risk on the part of powerful social actors, mainly those attracted to environmental causes. Their radicalism and allegiance from the unreflexive masses was allowed to grow, they argue, because of the 'softness' of core institutions, read the Catholic Church, in failing to condemn them. Although Lash rejects the inherent structural functionalist conservatism of Douglas and Wildavsky, he enthusiastically appropriates their idea of the sect and the subjective interpretation of risk, albeit with a positive twist, to suggest that such groups or sects are better conceptualised as anti-institutional because they are 'constructed in the context of institutional uncertainty of risk' (Lash 2002: 60) and may work to signal to others where such risks are located. Without hierarchy, sects comprise individuals who meld through mutual affection and intense commitment to common causes. Sects are possible because people join with others in their mutual incomplete and unfinished subjectivities; they define themselves in terms of lack rather than a certainty afforded through institutional traditions or rationality. As communities of affect, Lash (2002: 60) argues, sects espouse *values* rather than norms:

The sort of sociations that make up the critical risk cultures of reflexive modernity are not normative but value groupings that operate in the margins, in the third space, the boundary that separates private and public life. They are cultures and not institutions in the sense that they operate in the media of values not norms. But they are characteristically risk cultures . . . in that there is chronic uncertainty, a continual questioning, an openness to innovation built into them. They deal with risk, with identity-risks and ecological risks, not so much through rational calculation or normative subsumption, but through symbolic practises and especially through symbol innovation.

The significance of sects for Lash is that they represent a cultural vehicle in redefining realist interpretations of risk. In this enterprise, Lash invokes Kant's concept of reflexive judgement that emanates, not from rules of logic (determinate judgement), but from feelings. It takes place, not through understanding (cognitive, self-monitoring processes) of a priori rules, but through imagination and sensation. Reflexive judgement does not follow rules, it must look for rules; it is created, not logically, but 'through the approximation of "configurations" to one another' and then in synthesising or constructing new meanings (Lash 2002: 55). In a post-industrial milieu (as opposed to Beck's industrial risk society where risk is conceived as fixed, objectivist, norm-based and rationally defended) reflexive modernity comprises dynamic, anti-institutional, subjective and affective-based risk cultures.

The notion of constructed risk and risk cultures as comprising anti-institutional and critical but reflexive communities forged through affect and utilising reflexive judgement are useful propositions in attempting to unravel the complexities that surround the 'postmodernisation' of health care and the fast growing normalisation of CAM use, particularly by primary practitioners, such as general practitioners (GPs) (Eastwood 2000; Easthope et al. 2001; Rayner and Easthope 2001), nurses and midwives. The concept of risk culture promotes a more incisive understanding of the position of midwifery in appropriating CAM in primary care and in midwives repositioning themselves *vis-à-vis* obstetrics in the new collaborative care regime promoted by the post-welfare neoliberal state in Australia and elsewhere (Department of Human Services 2004).

The postmodernisation of health care: the emergence of risk cultures

Connor (2004) surmises from her study of residents of a small suburb in Australia that people use CAM therapies, in conjunction with other medicines, as a defensive strategy against the humanly manufactured risks of 'risk society'. Such risks include the lack of work/life balance, use of addictive substances and pollution of the natural world by the side-effects of industrialisation. Connor's study comprising 34 respondents (18 women, 14 men and 2 children) compares with other work that reports usage rates for men and women on a broader scale (Adams et al. 2003; Murray and Shepherd 1993) and an international review that found rates varied from 9% to 65% (Ernst 2000). Australian government surveys show that 42% of Australians use CAM treatments and similar findings have been made in the USA and the UK (Murray and Shepherd 1993; Eisenberg et al. 1998; Bensoussan 1999; Coulter and Willis 2004). An important next question is: why do significant numbers of people increasingly use CAM?

A somewhat surprising outcome of the rising use of CAM has been an increasing willingness on the part of allopathic practitioners (given their pronounced aversion to CAM) to at least consider the possible benefits or at least refer patients on to alternative practitioners. Many GPs have even undertaken short courses on some of the more popular options, such as meditation, relaxation therapies, herbal medicine, nutritional medicine, acupuncture, manipulation and homeopathy and have incorporated them into their own practice (Adams 2004; Eastwood 2000). Even the Australian Medical Association (2002) has been pressured by a groundswell within their own ranks to recognise the growth of interest among GPs but also among specialties such as obstetrics, gynaecology and rheumatology and to note an increasing demand on hospitals and pharmacies to produce policies in response to patients who desire continued use of CAM during hospitalisation. Of course this may signal, not an acceptance of the verities of CAM, but more a begrudging acknowledgement of its burgeoning use and an overarching concern to contain CAM within orthodox boundaries via standardisation, research evaluation, professional accreditation, regulation of practitioners and training for members.

The individualisation of risk

We need to account for the inevitable event that all information, including CAM discourses, are culturally mediated or selectively interpreted and used. Goldner (2004) intimated this by calling CAM a social movement because users comprise loose social networks through the sharing of information to create an alternative way of life. This is a useful step forward in understanding the political tendencies of CAM users. Many users identified by Goldner (2004) seek more 'balance' in their lives even when disease is not present; alternatively, those afflicted seek to improve their lives 'spiritually, emotionally, mentally and socially' (Goldner 2004: 15). The 'postmodernisation' of health care goes some way in explaining the rise of CAM (i.e. that users reject the legitimate authority of science and allopathy) but we also need to account for its momentum – that is, the increased acceptance among health consumers that health is an individual responsibility. The users in Goldner's (2004) study are a case in point. They were less concerned about the absence of scientific rationale than they were in practical efficacy; CAM empowered them to take individual responsibility for their health. Although these consumers did not believe they created the problem, they did believe that they were responsible for finding the solution.

This is where we might usefully employ Lash's (2002) concept of 'risk culture' or 'reflexive community' to explicate the growing use of CAM because 'risk culture' implies the individualisation of risk as well as a rejection of realist interpretations of risk and the body. At the very least, CAM users are placing 'a bet each way' on CAM and orthodox medicine (Bakx 1991; Siahpush 1999; Willis and White 2004). Users are not especially concerned that CAM lacks an objective, scientific, evidence-based grounding but follow a Kantian assessment that rejects the rules of logic (determinate judgement) in favour of feelings, imagination and sensation. So long as they believe that CAM gives them 'balance' users are not especially concerned with explaining how it works. Such reflexive judgement juxtaposes experiential knowledge to create new paradigms. As Goldner (2004) showed in her study of CAM users, respondents' activism began with positive results from which they embraced the foundational philosophies then projected their worldview into political campaigns whether these were individual-based or collective strategies. In rejecting the authenticity of orthodox biomedicine, CAM cultures signify via symbolic means (vital forces, energy fields, qui, chakras, spirit) where risks are located (neo-liberalism, capitalism, corporatised medicine, globalised pharmaceutical industries). CAM users are often passionate about their own health and see their own micro-interactions in terms of a macro-political framework where CAM is consistent with defending and healing an increasingly fragile universe.

The happy marriage of midwifery and CAM

The second part of my argument is that risk cultures can be applied fruitfully to understand a close affinity between CAM and midwifery. CAM refers generally to a diversity of practices and traditions that may be categorised broadly as those that adopt vitalistic principles at the centre of the healing modality. Vitalism conveys the understanding that any form of life is energised by a life-force that is more than the sum total of chemical and physical forces (Coulter 2004). Disease is said to be an outcome of the imbalance of the body's vital force caused by the interaction between the individual and the environment, including the social environment. This Kantian dialogic relationship between nature and culture produces a different set of assumptions about the relationship between practitioner and patient and a different approach to treatment. In assuming that both are active interpreters of the social environment, CAM promotes a more egalitarian exchange between equals at the heart of the clinical encounter. Treatment regimes are similarly sympathetic to the integrity of the individual body. Homeopathic remedies, for example, treat 'like with like' or, in other words, try to match the remedy with the symptoms of the disease on the grounds that the body will produce its own antidote. The medicine is used only to prompt a 'natural' recovery towards what they believe is a natural equilibrium. Biomedicine, by contrast, explains disease by reference to material causes. Cartesian dualism between mind and body, subject versus object, practitioner versus patient produces a hierarchical relationship between expert and (passive) recipient and with it a definition of illness as a malfunction of a particular body part (Coulter and Willis 2004; Collyer 2004). It follows that CAM and at least some midwifery practitioners will share intrinsic affinities that prove fortuitous in the shift towards consumerism under neoliberal political and economic reforms and individualisation under risk society or risk cultures.

'Realised' and 'latent' risk cultures: CAM use by midwives and the push of consumerism

Midwifery practice has traditionally occupied a strident binary opposition to obstetrics. This traditional dichotomy between techno-rationality and holism, however, has been ameliorated in more recent times by the collective forces of marketisation, managerialism and consumerism. In the push for value-for-money alternatives, neoliberal government policies have urged greater collaboration among midwives and obstetricians (Department of Health 2004; Reiger 2006) resulting in a blurring of professional boundaries and at least a limited convergence of ideas around childbirth practices (Lane 2006). It is now more useful to consider practitioners from both professions as occupying fluid positions along a sliding scale demarcated by a reductionist model of birth, the body and risk at one end of the continuum and a holistic model at the other. Individual positioning is neither entirely predictable nor static and will depend on a range of factors including: the place of birth (private versus public sector or home); the training and expertise of the midwife and obstetrician; the educational level and express wishes of the mother; and the perceived nature of the risk. Such complexities signify a greater degree of heterogeneity of practices now than in the past within midwifery and in medicine in defining and assessing risk and in providing optimal care for women (Lane 2002; 2006).

Notwithstanding individual differences in practices, significant differences remain in the respective spheres of practice of obstetrics and midwifery and in their assessment of risk. Midwives claim that 'woman-centred care' (as opposed to profession- or provider-centred care) optimally delivered via continuity of care by a known midwife is *the* antidote to adverse outcomes principally because it recognises individual choice and intrinsically works *with* the idiosyncratic needs of women, especially in labour and childbirth. Midwives describe their practice as comprising skilled techniques in calming, encouraging, facilitating, listening, looking for cues, anticipating needs and strengthening women's resolve to birth without intervention (Leap 2000). In assuming no differentiation between mind and body, this brand of holism is based upon providing a secure, peaceful and predictable environment where harmony between the woman and her social environment (and especially the carer) is the key to non-medical interventionist outcomes. Midwives claim that obstetrics, by contrast, is rule-governed and non-consumer-centric because the biomedical default position assumes that all births are potentially high-risk events. Logically, therefore, the obstetrician aligns with the baby to circumnavigate the primary risk variable that is the mother and her inherently risky body. Although many obstetricians now expect, and even welcome, women's demands for more information and choices (Lane 2006), they nevertheless draw the line much earlier on what is deemed 'safe'. The outcome is much higher rates of all kinds of interventions under obstetric care sometimes referred to as the 'cascade of intervention' (foetal heart monitoring, syntocinin augmentation to speed up labour, epidural, forceps extraction, episiotomy and caesarean section). Ironically, obstetricians say they use these procedures to anticipate risk before it occurs (Lane 2006).

The irony is that from a holistic, midwifery paradigm the positivist mindset, rather than the mother's inept body, represents the most potent site of risk (Lane 1995). For holistic midwifery practitioners the key to safe practise is the Kantian dialogical relationship between practitioner and patient (Collyer 2004) – that is, relations based upon mutual respect, integrity and reciprocity (Lane 2000). The commensurability between CAM and midwifery is that both require patients to extensively discuss their idiosyncratic location in the world for the optimal medicine to be prescribed. This is what midwifery means when describing its practice as 'with women' (Leap and Hunter 1993). The idea that the relationship is actually a 'partnership' (Guilliland and Pairman 1995) is now an accepted part of the lexicon of midwifery practice (*Victorian Midwifery Code of Practice*, Nurses Board of Victoria 1999) appearing in leading midwifery training texts:

> A midwife forms a partnership with a woman as she experiences the life process of childbearing and early parenting. Midwifery care is woman-centred . . . The midwife shares knowledge, experience and wisdom reciprocally with the woman and her family. The midwife protects and promotes the dignity of each woman and accepts her culture, beliefs, values, expectations and previous experiences. The midwife and the woman make decisions together through a process of negotiation.
>
> (Pairman et al. 2006: vii)

Holistic care, 'woman-centred' practice and 'continuity of care' constitute key features that midwives claim distinguish their practice from obstetrics. The latter is based more on a defensive style of care, a 'just in case' syndrome, that encourages a greater use of technology and thus restricts choices for women. Conversely, 'best practice' midwifery is defined as woman centred, rather than profession or institution centred. It is on this premise that one recent training manual (Tiran and Mack 2000: 6–11) promotes the use of complementary therapies (massage, relaxation, meditation, visualisation, guided imagery, play and humour, music, therapeutic touch and a healing environment in pregnancy and childbirth) as ideal modalities to achieve increased choice and control for women, a better emotional experience and a safe delivery without unwanted side-effects for the mother or her baby:

> [Complementary therapies have] . . . fewer side-effects than many of the pharmaceutical options, and enable the mother to achieve not only a

safe delivery of a healthy child but also to experience a satisfying, significant episode in her life. Mothers and midwives are looking to complementary therapies to avoid the risks of drugs to the unborn baby . . . provide more natural advice for the relief of common discomforts of pregnancy and the postnatal period and [provide] . . . alternative forms of pain relief in labour.

(Tiran and Mack 2000: 10–11)

Significantly, this manual suggests CAM is to be used in consultation with the client who no longer accepts the belief that 'doctor knows best' or that allopathic medicine has all the answers (Tiran and Mack 2000: 3–4):

while orthodox medicine views the body in a reductionist manner, as an engine which can be dismantled, mended and reassembled, irrespective of temperament, personality, emotions or external influences, CAM is based on an understanding of the interaction between body, mind and spirit, and a recognition of each person as an individual in the wider context of the environment.

Further, CAM 'expands choices for women and helps them to feel in control of their own wellbeing' (Tiran and Mack 2000: 3–4). The fact that CAM therapies lack scientific support should not deter midwives from using them, it is stated, because the randomised, double-blind controlled clinical trial is 'not always an appropriate methodology for complementary medical research' (Tiran and Mack 2000: 5). For these authors, CAM and midwifery are perfect partners in providing optimal health care for women. Both harbour philosophies that reject biomedical reductionism and both regard individuals as reflexive subjects whose symptoms mirror their discrete interpretation of a complex environment where choice and active involvement are fundamental requisites in the healing process; both therefore are holistic and see healing as more 'art than science' (May and Sirur 1998). But can we regard midwifery as properly coming under a 'CAM risk culture'?

Despite the obvious convergences between CAM and midwifery, there is little indication that midwifery political bodies or mainstream educational curricula have embraced CAM usage as a natural ally of consumer choice and continuity-of-care. The Australian College of Midwifery Inc. has posted no position statement on CAM (unlike the Australian Medical Association [AMA]) and a recent text on midwifery practice (Pairman et al. 2006) specifically avoids discussion of CAM usage by midwives except briefly to caution undergraduates that the efficacy of CAM for pain or discomfort is yet to be proven. Midwives were warned not to assume that 'natural' or 'alternative' means 'safer, lower risk or more effective than conventional options'. Rather than promoting CAM remedies, midwives were urged to advise their clients to adopt a healthy lifestyle, healthy diet and follow a moderate exercise regime (Grigg 2006: 366). However, Lash (2002) argues that risk cultures are by definition marginal. Building on this, we might distinguish between *latent* and *realised* risk cultures. CAM sympathisers within midwifery who are usually community-based independent midwives could be called a *realised* risk culture in that they espouse egalitarian, holistic values, are reflexively interpretive and judiciously anti-science. While mainstream midwifery practised in hospitals is dominated by obstetric protocols, it may still be regarded as anti-institutional in relation to the objectivist mindset of obstetrics. All midwifery practice sees risk in intervening too early in a woman's labour, in imposing standardised timeframes in which the woman must progress through labour and in undermining her confidence in her ability to give birth without drugs and surgical procedures. Thus all midwives constitute, at least notionally, a *latent* risk culture.

Individualisation

It is necessary at this point to take a detour to Beck and Beck-Gernsheim's (2002) concept of individualisation or, 'institutionalised individualism' which points, like the 'Risk Society' thesis (Beck 1992), to a new epoch of modernity called second modernity or reflexive modernity. Individualisation is the flip side of the Risk Society; it refers, not to the neoliberal idea of the self-sufficient individual and the disappearance of mutual obligation, but to the fundamental incompleteness of the self. In developed modernity, the central institutions protecting civil, political and economic rights, including the labour market, education and health, are geared towards the individual. Giddens (1992) called this the 'disembedding of social relations' whereas Beck and Beck-Gernsheim (2002) call it 'individualisation' meaning 'an institutionalised imbalance between the disembedded individual and global problems in a global risk society' (Beck and Beck-Gernsheim 2002: xxi–xxii). Individualisation refers not to a 'me-first' society, but an 'ideal intimacy situation' (borrowing from Habermas) that governs the construction of specific rules for intimate, reciprocal interactions. The old structures – class, gender, ethnicity and status – no longer mould the individual. Rather, the individual is shaped by an ethic of self-fulfilment and achievement. It is a search for a 'life of one's own in a runaway world' (Beck and Beck-Gernsheim 2002: 22–9); an attempt at social cohesion when the new ontologies of Western culture are formed from individualism, diversity and scepticism. Individuals are forced to be free to construct their own biographies, including their own failures, and their own traditions. They must be reflexive – to be able to process contradictory discourses within the risk society of global uncertainty.

Individualisation has transformed the concept of health and the body from the idea of having 'lucky genes' to a task, an ongoing project and a life achievement and to this end a reflexive individual will visit a variety of modalities and, more significantly, actively institute ways to prevent illness via a 'proper' lifestyle, diet, exercise and life choices and probably above all a positive mindset. Under individualisation, health infers, not the absence of illness, but a vehicle to optimal personal performance.

CAM and autonomous professional practice

It is my thesis that, potentially at least, CAM provides a fortuitous crux to the emergence of the midwife as primary carer at a time when the neoliberal state is encouraging the dissolution of professional boundaries that may impede economic efficiencies. The National Competency Standards for the Midwife (ANMC 2002), for example, defines the midwife as:

> a responsible and accountable professional who works in partnership with women to give the necessary support, care and advice during pregnancy, labour and the postpartum period, to conduct births *on the midwife's own responsibility* and to provide care for the newborn and the infant. This care includes preventative measures, the promotion of normal birth, the detection of complications in mother and child, the accessing of medical care or other appropriate assistance and the carrying out of emergency measures . . . A midwife may practise in any setting including the home, community, hospitals, clinics or health units.
> (ANMC 2002: 1; emphasis added)

The history of midwifery subordination

These internationally agreed upon dictums demand the midwife be professionally autonomous. Specifically she/he should carry out preventive treatment and only as a last resort call for medical assistance. In practice, such autonomy has been vastly undermined by legal regulations and obstetric and hospital protocols that had been transplanted from the British medical system and instituted within Australia at the time of early settlement (Willis 1983).

Legal control of midwifery in Australia is now variously apportioned in different statutes and regulations in each of the states. The Victorian and Tasmanian statutes have been the most repressive. Tasmanian regulations stipulated that women must attend a medical practice for maternity care and 1985 Victorian Midwifery Regulations 601–604 propped up obstetric dominance by requiring medical supervision of all midwifery activity, including vaginal examinations, manipulative procedures and delivery. Unsurprisingly, consumer and midwifery calls for the abolition of the regulations were thwarted by the College of Obstetricians and Gynaecologists. These kinds of legal constraints on autonomous midwifery gradually diminished in light of recommendations made by government reviews of birthing services in most states in the 1990s. These recommendations included a more active role for midwives in and outside of hospitals, the public funding of community (homebirth) midwifery (only now being considered), the development of a direct entry midwifery degree (which has now eventuated fifteen years later), the recognition of overseas trained direct entry midwives (normally from the Netherlands or Britain), and the granting of hospital visiting rights for independently practising midwives (Deptartment of Health Victoria 1990: 155–6).

Some state governments (Victoria, New South Wales and Northern Territory) have more recently recognised the cost savings to be achieved under caseload models that ensure that women receive one-on-one care throughout their maternity careers by a known midwife (Reiger 2006). This is an important shift not just in midwifery autonomy but in achieving better outcomes for women because evidence suggests that continuity of care by a known midwifery is *the* best assurance of lower intervention rates and lower rates of morbidity (and lower costs) (Oakley and Houd 1990).

The one remaining obstacle to full autonomy for midwifery, at least technically, has been the removal of professional indemnity insurance in the aftermath of the collapse of HIH (Heath International Holdings) although there are encouraging signs recently that one insurer is finally prepared to provide professional indemnity for all midwives regardless of where they practise.[1] This may encourage the expansion of autonomy although residual cultural factors pose the greatest barriers. These include the consequences of decades of deskilling under labour-force deployments where midwives were assigned exclusively to one of three areas of maternity care – antenatal, delivery and postnatal units. This fragmentation effectively divided midwifery into specialties and downgraded them as obstetric assistants. The outcome has been depleted skills and a correspondingly deflated midwifery identity among the majority of midwives, but particularly those who work in hospitals. The upshot of such developments is that few midwives are currently willing to volunteer to take on the caseload mantle although this may change when graduates from current Bachelor of Midwifery (direct entry) courses in South Australia, Victoria and New South Wales make their presence felt in large enough numbers in the labour-force. There are early signs that a new professionalism is emerging – one that encourages midwives to regard themselves as fully autonomous professionals in partnership with both obstetricians and women in the delivery of maternity care (Lane 2006).

In terms of risk assessment, qualitative and quantitative studies have shown that obstetric care in hospitals has never been safer than delivery at home attended by a midwife (Tew 1990), although such claims can only be authenticated if there is an adequately skilled midwifery workforce. CAM may yet prove instrumental in promoting the caseload model as it propels the midwife into the role of primary carer and autonomous professional. The Australian College of Holistic Nurses endorses the signal advantage of CAM interventions because it protects midwifery autonomy: 'carried out within the scope of nursing or midwifery practice [CAM therapies] do not require a medical practitioner's order' (Australian College of Holistic Nurses 2002: 6–7). Of course other practitioners (complementary/alternative therapist, pharmacist, medical practitioner) may be consulted but only when circumstances dictate. Although primary health care has traditionally been the province of general practice (Dowell and Neal 2000: 9) its holistic parameters could equally describe the increasing role of one-to-one, caseload midwifery with its 'value-for-money' qualities (Power 1999), including the substitution of expensive obstetric care, 24-hour personal and family care and its potential to realise lower medical interventions. In short, CAM has attractive qualities in realising midwifery autonomy.

The transformative integration pattern of medicine

Collyer (2004) has argued that CAM expansionism has been driven by commercial opportunism which is slowly transforming its cottage industry status into corporatisation. Although CAM has been mainstreamed, what arises (according to CAM practitioners) through a superficial merging of treatment regimes on the basis of a short introduction, is a loss of the philosophical basis of holism and a dilution of the healing potential. Kailin (2001 in Coulter 2004) has argued that attempts to integrate biomedicine with natural medicine often fall short of the objectives of all stakeholders. Allopathic practitioners typically contain CAM by imposing a biomedical perspective on the disease and employing CAM in a limited way within their own paradigm (Adams 2004). Consumers lose because the medicine is imposed uniformly according to surface symptoms rather than applied sensitively according to their unique constitutional disposition and complex causes. Nevertheless, one option is the 'transformative integration pattern' (Coulter 2004). Here CAM and biomedicine mutually inform each other within a close collegial relationship. The question is whether this kind of respectful relationship between medicine and CAM is likely to emerge within maternity care.

The issue is best represented as a battle between dominant and marginal discourses. The AMA requires hard evidence from double-blind randomised controlled trials (RCTs) to ensure CAM medicines pass the three pillars test – safety, quality and efficacy (AMA 2002). The problem is that CAM remedies are not easily evaluated by randomised controlled trials (Pirotta 2006). The assumption underlying the RCT is that patients are the same – that the body is a universal, uniform mechanism (Dew 2002). However, modalities such as homeopathy are based upon the opposite premise that one's constitution is a complex amalgam of life experiences that renders the universal body an impossible concept. In an experiment, the body cannot be kept constant so that differential outcomes test the intervention. Indeed, one of the challenges for the holistic practitioner is to ascertain exactly each patient's constitution to prescribe exactly the right medicine and this may only be achieved through a very long, in-depth interview. Even then after following such detailed inquiry, finding the right medicine is trial and error due to the complexity of individual identity.

Extrapolating a view of the body and identity as complex entities explains why midwives generally define risk in childbirth as precipitous medical intervention; their critique of obstetrics is that it pathologises the normal (Lane 2006). Normal birth may occur outside predetermined timeframes because individuals labour at different rates and treatments are determined by individual responses to their immediate social environment, medical and obstetric history and idiosyncratic choice. Midwives claim their practice is premised on birth as a normal, physiological process and significant life event (ANMC 2002) where each woman will require different types of assistance depending on how she constructs her life's narrative. The sociological adage that biography becomes biology is nowhere more evident than in childbirth. By conceptualising birth as a social event that requires idiosyncratic social support rather than medical interventions, midwives are more likely to adopt CAM within the realm of preventive care when appropriate and always in consultation with the woman. This philosophy constitutes the use of CAM within a 'transformative integration pattern' – transformative (of the old hierarchical relations) due to the refusal to compromise holistic principles and only for use in consultation with the woman.

Conclusion

I have argued in this chapter that we need to take a constructionist view of risk. Risk is anticipated by different cultures differently; risks are attached to situated knowledge (Haraway 1988). Lash (2002) proposes that we abandon the idea of risk society (a realist objectivist notion of risk) in favour of risk cultures. Risk cultures define themselves not in terms of rules of logic but in terms of reflexive judgement drawn from imagination and sensation. In a post-industrial milieu, risk is not fixed, norm-based and rationally defended, but dynamic, anti-institutional, subjective and affective-based. I have argued that CAM users and practitioners may be usefully categorised under this banner. They eschew rational scientific philosophies in favour of holism, vitalism and naturalism (Coulter 2004). Midwives may not universally advocate the use of CAM remedies. However, I argue that CAM has two distinct advantages for midwives. First, CAM allows midwives to galvanise their 'partnership' relationship with women. This is an organic relationship because 'partnership' defines midwifery profession-alism and practice and thus CAM can only strengthen such a relationship. Second, CAM is consistent with holistic midwifery practice and the quest for autonomy (from obstetrics) because both CAM and holism lie outside of medical positivism and reductionism. As such CAM and midwifery are natural allies. Finally, in line with these themes, there appears every likeli-hood that CAM use would be executed by midwives in a transformative way – that is, in the quest for an integrative model of care that refused to sacrifice holism or active consumer participation.

Note

1 Contracting Advantage offers two operating systems:

1 The ODCO System – Agency services to hospitals and other establishments with permanent employees.
2 Independent System – Agency services on a user pays basis for self-employed contractors.

The ODCO Pty Ltd System: This is the original contracting system set up for self-employed contractors. The system has been tested in courts several times and has been legitimised after Unions questioned the legality of the Agency. The ODCO system continues providing services for contractors, is audited and complies with the legal requirement of appropriate Licensing Boards. An example of the ODCO System working for a Private Midwifery Practice: If the company Melbourne Midwifery wanted to permanently employ full-time or part-time midwives, the ODCO system would require a 10% Administration fee; 5% paid by Melbourne Midwifery and 5% by each employed midwife. This system can be offered with cost savings to hospitals, universities and other organisations employing full- or part-time midwives. A midwife who both has private clients and is employed by a hospital system must be clear in declaring her/his client contractual arrangements from the outset.

The Independent System: In this case a user pay system provides individual access for midwives to Professional Indemnity and Public Liability Insurance for any sphere of practice – antenatal, labour and birth, postnatal, education (inside or outside hospital settings). The system is flexible – it will meet the needs of midwives who have not yet set up a business and for those who have well-established business facilities. Midwives pay a $500 per year up front fee for the Insurance Policy; there are no professional or other exclusions. The ACMI Codes and Guidelines are used for risk assessment. The back-end Admin-istration is similar for both Systems; CAdv can deal with invoicing clients on behalf of midwives, or midwives in established businesses can choose to continue without disruption their individual accounting and payment systems.

(Broadcast email to Maternity Coalition members from R. Thompson, Director, Melbourne Midwifery Pty Ltd, 6 September 2006).

References

ACHN (Australian College of Holistic Nurses) (2002) *Policy Guidelines for Practice of Complementary Therapies by Nurses and Midwives in Australia*, November. Brisbane: ACHN.

Adam, B. and van Loon, J. (2002) Introduction: Repositioning risk: the challenge for social theory. In Adam, B., Beck, U. and Van Loon, J. (eds) *The Risk Society and Beyond: Critical Issues for Social Theory.* London: Sage, pp. 1–32.

Adams, J. (2004) Demarcating the medical/non-medical border: occupational boundary-work within GPs' accounts of their integrative practice. In Tovey, P., Easthope, G. and Adams, J. (eds) *The Mainstreaming of Complementary and Alternative Medicine: Studies in Social Context.* London: Routledge, pp. 140–57.

Adams, J., Sibbritt, D., Easthope, G. and Young, A. (2003) The profile of women who consult alternative health practitioners in Australia. *Medical Journal of Australia* 179(6): 297–300.

AMA (Australian Medical Association) (2002) *Position Statement on Complementary Medicine*: http://www.ama.com.au

ANMC (Australian Nursing and Midwifery Council) (2002) *National Competency Standards for the Midwife.* Dickson, ACT: ANMC.

Bakx, K. (1991) The 'eclipse' of folk medicine in Western society. *Sociology of Health and Illness* 13: 20–39.

Beck, U. (1992) *Risk Society: Towards a New Modernity.* London, Sage.

Beck, U. and Beck-Gernsheim, E. (2002) *Individualisation.* London, Sage.

Beck, U., Giddens, A. and Lash, S. (1994) *Reflexive Modernisation.* Cambridge: Polity Press.

Bensoussan, A. (1999) Complementary medicine – where lies its appeal? *Medical Journal of Australia* 170: 247–8.

Blackmore, J. and Sachs, J. (2007) *Performing and Reforming Leaders: Gender, Educational Restructuring and Organizational Change.* New York: SUNY Press.

Clark, A., Shim, J. K., Mano, L., Forsket, J. R. and Fishman, J. R. (2003) Biomedicalisation: technoscientific transformations of health, illness and US biomedicine. *American Sociological Review* 66: 161–94.

Collyer, F.. (2004) The corporatisation and commercialisation of CAM. In Tovey, P., Easthope, G. and Adams, J. (eds) *The Mainstreaming of Complementary and Alternative Medicine, Studies in Social Context.* London and New York: Routledge, pp. 81–102.

Connor, L. H. (2004) Relief, risk and renewal: mixed therapy regimens in an Australian suburb. *Social Science & Medicine* 59(8): 1695–705.

Coulter, I. (2004) Integration and paradigm clash: the practical difficulties of integrative medicine. In Tovey, P., Easthope, G. and Adams, J. (eds) *The Mainstreaming of Complementary and Alternative Medicine, Studies in Social Context.* London and New York: Routledge, pp. 103–22.

Coulter, I. D. and Willis, E. M. (2004) The rise and rise of complementary and alternative medicine: a sociological perspective. *The Medical Journal of Australia* 180(11): 587–9.

Department of Health Victoria (1990) *Final Report of the Ministerial Review of Birthing Services in Victoria: Having a Baby in Victoria* (Birthing Services Review). Melbourne: Department of Health Victoria.

Department of Human Services (2004) *New Directions in Maternity Care*. Victoria: Department of Human Services.

Dew, K. (2002) The regulation of practice: practitioners and their interactions with organisations. In Tovey, P., Easthope, G. and Adams, J. (eds) *The Mainstreaming of Complementary and Alternative Medicine: Studies in Social Context*. London and New York: Routledge, pp. 64–80.

Douglas, M. and Wildavsky, A. (1983) *Risk and Culture*, Berkeley, CA: University of California Press.

Dowell, T. and Neal, R. (2000) Vision and change in primary care: past, present and future. In Tovey, P. (ed.) *Contemporary Primary Care: The Challenges of Change*. Buckingham: Open University Press, pp. 9–25.

Easthope, G. (2004) Consuming health: the market for complementary and alternative medicine. *Australian Journal of Primary Health* 10(2): 68–75.

Easthope, G., Tranter, B. and Gill, G. (2001) The incorporation of a complementary therapy by Australian general practitioners: the case of acupuncture. *Australian Journal of Primary Health* 7(1): 76–81.

Eastwood, H. (2000) Why are Australian GPs using alternative medicine? Post-modernisation, consumerism and the shift towards holistic health. *Journal of Sociology* 36(2): 133–56.

Eisenberg, D. M., Davis, R. B. and Ettner, S. L. (1998) Trends in alternative medicine use in the United States. *Journal of the American Medical Association* 280: 1569–75.

Ernst, E. (2000) Prevalence of use of complementary/alternative medicine: a systematic review. *Bulletin of the World Health Organization* 78(2): 252–7.

Giddens, A. (1992) *The Transformation of Intimacy*. Cambridge: Polity Press.

Goldner, M. (2004) Consumption as activism: an examination of CAM as part of the consumer movement in health. In Tovey, P., Easthope, G. and Adams, J. (eds) *The Mainstreaming of Complementary and Alternative Medicine: Studies in Social Context*. London and New York: Routledge, pp. 11–24.

Grigg, C. (2006) Working with women in pregnancy. In Pairman S., Pincombe J., Thorogood C., Tracy S., *Midwifery: Preparation for Practice*. Sydney: Elsevier, pp. 341–73.

Guililand, K. and Pairman, S. (1995) *The Midwifery Partnership: A Model for Practice*. Department of Nursing and Midwifery, Monograph Series 95/1, Victoria University of Wellington, Wellington.

Haraway, D. (1988) Situated knowledges: the sciences question in feminism and the privilege of partial perspective. *Feminist Studies* 14(3): 575–99.

Kailin, D. C. (2001) Initial strategies. In Faass, N. (ed) *Integrating Complementary Medicine into Health Systems*. Gaithersburg, MD: Aspen Publishers, pp. 44–58.

Lane, K. (1995) The medical model of the body as a site of risk: a case study of childbirth. In Gabe, J. (ed.) *Medicine, Health and Risk: Sociological Approaches*, Sociology of Health and Illness Monograph Series. Oxford: Blackwell, pp. 53–72.

Lane, K. (2000) Consumers as arbiters of professional practice? What does this mean for users of maternity services? *Sociological Sites/Sights: TASA 2000 Conference*: 1–8.

Lane, K. (2002) Midwifery: a profession in transition. *Australian Journal of Midwifery* 15(2): 26–31.

Lane, K. (2006) The plasticity of professional boundaries: a case study of collaborative care in maternity services. *Health Sociology Review* 15(4): 341–52.

Lash, S. (2002) Risk culture. In Adam, B., Beck, U. and van Loon, J. (eds) *The Risk Society and Beyond: Critical Issues for Social Theory*. London: Sage, pp. 47–62.

Leap, N. (2000) The less we do the more we give. In Kirkham, M. (ed.) *The Midwife/Mother Relationship*. Hants: Palgrave Macmillan, pp. 74–85.

Leap, N. and Hunter, B. (1993) *The Midwife's Tale: An Oral History from Handywoman to Professional Midwife*. Gateshead: Scarlet Press.

May, C. and Sirur, D. (1998) Art, science and placebo: incorporating homeopathy in general practice. *Sociology of Health and Illness* 20(2): 168–90.

Murray, J. and Shepherd, S. (1993) Alternative or additional medicine? An exploratory study in general practice. *Social Science & Medicine* 37(8): 983–8.

Nurses Board of Victoria (1999) Victorian Midwifery Code of Practice. Melbourne: Nurses Board of Victoria.

Oakley, A. and Houd, S. (1990) Who is at risk? In Oakley, A. and Houd, S. (eds) *Helpers in Childbirth: Midwifery Today*. New York: Hemisphere Publishing Corporation, pp. 115–31.

Pairman, S., Pincombe, J., Thorogood, C. and Tracy, S. (2006) *Midwifery: Preparation for Practice*. Sydney: Elsevier.

Pirotta, M. (2006) Towards the application of RCTs for CAM: methodological challenges. In Adams, J. (ed.) *Researching Complementary and Alternative Medicine*. London: Routledge, pp. 52–71.

Power, M. (1999) *The Audit Society: Rituals of Verification*. Oxford: Oxford University Press.

Rayner, L. and Easthope, G. (2001) Postmodern consumption and alternative medications. *Journal of Sociology*, Australian Sociological Association, 37(2): 157–76.

Reiger, K. (2006) A Neo-liberal quickstep: contradictions in Australian maternity policy. *Health Sociology Review*, ed. Reiger, K., Possamei-Inesedy, A. and Lane, K., October, Special Birth Edition: 330–40.

Scott, A. (2002) Two views of risk, consciousness and community. In Adam, B., Beck, U. and van Loon, J. (eds) *The Risk Society and Beyond: Critical Issues for Social Theory*. London: Sage, pp. 33–46.

Siahpush, M. (1999) Why do people favour alternative medicine? *Australia and New Zealand Journal of Public Health* 23: 266–71; 29: 289–301.

Skinner, J. (2006) Risk and safety. In Pairman, S., Pincombe, J., Thorogood, C. and Tracy, S. (eds) *Midwifery: Preparation for Practice*. Marrickville, NSW: Elsevier, pp. 61–71.

Tew, M. (1990) *Safer Childbirth? A Critical History of Maternity Care*. London: Chapman and Hall.

Tiran, D. and Mack, S. (2000) Incorporation of complementary therapies into maternity care. In Tiran, D. and Mack, S. (eds) *Complementary Therapies for Pregnancy and Childbirth*, 2nd edn. Edinburgh: Bailliere Tindall, pp. 1–15.

Willis, E. (1983) *Medical Dominance: The Division of Labour in Australian Health Care*. Sydney: George Allen and Unwin.

Willis, E. and White, K. (2004) Evidence-based medicine and CAM. In Tovey, P., Easthope, G. and Adams, J. (eds) *The Mainstreaming of Complementary and Alternative Medicine, Studies in Social Context*. London and New York: Routledge, pp. 49–63.

Chapter 8

CAM, holistic wellness nursing and the new public health

Emily Hansen

Introduction

Holistic wellness nursing is a nursing philosophy that stresses the importance of maintaining health, the 'whole person' and self-responsibility for health and well-being (Chambers-Clark 1986). Nurses practising the approach often utilise complementary and alternative medicine (CAM) treatment modalities for the purpose of disease prevention and health promotion (Plawecki 1996; Wong et al. 2001; Fenton and Morris 2003). In this chapter I establish areas of commonality between holistic wellness nursing and the new public health, and explore the relevance of the socio-cultural critique of the new public health for holistic wellness nursing.

Holistic wellness nursing

Holistic wellness nursing is a philosophy that promotes the integration, balance and harmony of 'mind and spirit', that emphasises 'the process of self healing rather than disease' and views illness as 'an opportunity for growth and increased self-awareness' (Boschma 1994: 324). The holistic nursing model emerged in the USA in the 1960s and 1970s (Allen 1991) and is now sufficiently established in the USA to support a professional nursing organisation named the American Holistic Nurses Association (which has released standards for holistic nursing practice), a large number of websites and a journal titled *Holistic Nursing Practice* (Baer 2004). Articles about holistic nursing are also published in other nursing journals such as *Public Health Nursing* and *Journal of Advanced Nursing* and several American nursing schools now specialise in a holistic nursing approach (King and Gates 2006; Frisch 2003). Units on holistic nursing are also offered in several North American nursing undergraduate courses and are being established in universities in countries such as Israel (Hoover 2002; Fenton and Morris 2003; Shuval 2006).

Wellness nursing is a sub-set of holistic nursing that focuses on 'healthy' people in an effort to increase their well-being and prevent illness in the future (Bacon et al. 2002; Drewnowski et al. 2003). Wellness is defined as 'a process of moving towards greater awareness of oneself and the environment leading toward ever increasing planned interactions with the dimensions of nutrition, fitness, stress, environment, interpersonal relationships and self care responsibility' (Chambers-Clark 1986: 3). Similar definitions of wellness are also found in physical education, counselling and education texts (Anspaugh et al. 1994; Greenberg et al. 1997; Lowdon et al. 1993). Despite the overt focus on maintaining and improving well-being, concepts of wellness do *not* exclude people with existing illness or those who are dying. Some wellness nurse practitioners emphasise the value of a wellness approach for patients with terminal or serious chronic conditions arguing that 'even though an individual may be dying of a physical ailment, that individual may be able to function at a high level of wellness' (Swinford and Webster 1989: 5). Articles about holistic nursing interventions show the approach being applied in a wide range of health-related situations in addition to health promotion and disease prevention. These include emergency room nursing, treating alcoholism, and caring for the elderly, burn victims and people affected by chronic illness (see, for example, Paul and Weinert 1999; Ford and McCormack 2000).

Holistic and wellness nursing philosophies emerged as part of the process of professionalisation by American nurses in the 1950s, 1960s and 1970s and with attempts to understand, explain, define and justify the role and contribution of nurses through the development of nursing theory (Allen 1991; Woods 1987; McCoppin and Gardner 1994; Baer 2004; Shuval 2006). Holistic ideas within nursing are associated with the hospice movement and palliative care nursing, the primary health care movement, feminist nursing, feminist and postmodern medical ethics and the increased use of the social sciences (in particular psychology) in nursing education (Petosa 1984; Chambers-Clark 1986; Johnson 1990; Hoffmann 1991; Siahpush 1998).

Holistic nursing is also closely linked with the 1960s holistic health movement (Boschma 1994: 325; Baer 2004) and associated with 1960s counterculture and social movements such as the civil rights movement, environmentalism, feminism and CAM and can be viewed as part of the 'larger context of disappointment with the effects of science and technology' (Boschma 1994: 328). Nurses have been attracted to holistic or wellness nursing because they are dissatisfied with biomedicine. For example, Auger describes personal disillusionment with 'official medical practices' as her motive for training as a holistic nurse (Auger 1990). Slater and colleagues reviewed phenomenological accounts of becoming a holistic nurse-practitioner and found that nurses described their attraction to a holistic nursing philosophy in terms of their desire for an approach that fostered self-care, that supported patients emotionally and spiritually and which involved 'the healing energy of love' (Slater et al. 1999: 381). Indeed, nurses more generally have been found to describe and justify their practices in contrast to the biomedical approach adopted by doctors (Adams 2006; Adams and Tovey 2001).

However, the claim that holistic nursing is a distinct nursing speciality is itself an area of debate and tension given the long held notion within nursing that *all* nurses should provide holistic care and have a holistic viewpoint (Boschma 1994; Pender 1982: 39). An understanding that nursing is a fundamentally holistic health care profession is closely linked with perceptions among nurses that caring, focusing on the whole person and a concern with patient interests are core traditional nursing values (Tovey and Adams 2003). Holistic nursing is also linked to patient-centred nursing models which require practitioners to view the patient as a 'whole person' and as an individual (Tovey and Adams 2003).

Due to links with the wider holistic health movement and thus the holistic philosophy that underpins many CAM modalities, holistic wellness nursing is strongly linked with CAM concepts and practices. While CAM is not essential to holistic or wellness nursing, nurses who identify themselves as holistic or wellness nurses appear more likely to use various types of CAM such as affirmations, guided imagery, energy healing, acupuncture, aromatherapy and therapeutic massage (Plawecki 1996; Giasson and Bouchard 1998; Cohen and Bumbaugh 2004; Helms 2006).

Holistic and wellness nursing textbooks frequently advise that nurses apply a range of alternative/holistic healing modalities. For example, Chambers-Clark (1986) recommends that nurses teach their clients the use of positive affirmations and positive imagery to help adopt and maintain healthy lifestyle practices, such as taking up exercise, or in order to give up unhealthy practices such as smoking. Plawecki (1996: 84) argues that 'describing, examining and investigating treatment modalities which are currently described as alternative' is one of the goals of holistic nursing. He also describes eastern philosophy, biofeedback, therapeutic and healing touch, aromatherapy, religion, spirituality and cultural beliefs as 'just a few of the topics that may directly influence the practice of holistic nursing' (1996: 83–4). Holistic and wellness nursing journal articles also describe the application of treatments or practices such as dreamwork, reiki, acupuncture and therapeutic touch (Fenton and Morris 2003; Zengerle-Levy 2004).

Holistic wellness nurses' use of CAM is not surprising. Holistic thinking shares many values with CAM such as viewing people as 'simultaneously biological and social creatures' and an emphasis on 'individuality, interpersonal interaction with patients, subjectivity of experience, feeling, self-healing, energy, balance and prevention' (Shuval 2006: 1785). Thus, CAM and holistic nursing are highly compatible, perhaps more so than holistic nursing and biomedicine. However, as Shuval and others have shown, nurses and doctors who use CAM are doing so as biomedically trained persons who view CAM as complementary rather than as an alternative to biomedicine (Cant and Sharma 2000; Adams 2004; Shuval 2006).

Holistic wellness nursing and the new public health

The new public health is a public health philosophy that emerged in the late 1970s and moved to prominence through the World Health Organization and State public health policy in countries like Canada, the United Kingdom and Australia by the late 1980s (Nettleton 1995: 232). Supporters of the new public health claim that it moves beyond a reductive biomedical view of health towards a broadly based biopsychosocial and environmental understanding of health and disease prevention. They argue that traditional public health emphasised hygiene, modern health promotion focuses almost entirely on lifestyle risk factor reduction and mainstream medical thinking (germ theory) emphasises the importance of medical care for health. In contrast, the new public health has a much broader and more general conception of the social aspects of disease. It emphasises that lifestyle, socio-economic factors, the environment and health care systems *all* play an important role in achieving and maintaining health. As O'Connor and Parker explain, 'what has emerged under the title of "new public health" is an approach that brings together environmental change and personal preventive measures with appropriate therapeutic interventions' (O'Connor and Parker 1995: 7). Ashton and Seymour describe the new public health as an approach where 'many contemporary health problems are therefore seen as social rather than solely individual problems' and where 'the environment is social and psychological as well as physical' (Aston and Seymour 1988: 21).

Thus, in theory, the new public health operates with a biopsychosocial understanding of health and requires education and lifestyle modification to be part of general public policy, the workplace and education. The new public health also claims to be directed not only to health issues in a narrow sense, but also to broader social, political, and economic conditions that produce differences in health among different groups. For example, the five strategies for health promotion outlined in the Ottawa Charter framework are: building healthy public policy; creating supportive environments; developing personal skills; strengthening community action; and reorientating health services (WHO 1986). It is important to point out, however, that while the new public health is broad ranging in theory, many writers argue that in application practitioners tend to fall back on reductive identification of risk factors in health promotion and lifestyle education campaigns.

Holistic wellness nursing and the new public health have several characteristics in common. First, they share an expanded health concept which is biopsychosocial (Lowenberg 1989). A biopsychosocial understanding of disease prevention and health maintenance means that the range and number of behaviours and practices viewed as being related to health (and requiring some type of medical advice or intervention) is dramatically increased. The meaning of these everyday behaviours and practices is changed because they are increasingly defined in terms of their relationship towards either damaging health, or promoting and maintaining good health (Fullagar 2002).

Wellness and holistic nursing have an even broader conception of health than those found in discourses of the new public health because they also draw on CAM discourses of health and well-being. For example, definitions of wellness include reference to factors such as environmental sensitivity, a joy in living, physical fitness, nutrition, healthful finances, occupational satisfaction, stress awareness and management (Ardell 1982; Petosa 1984).

Wellness nursing and the new public health both assume that health (or wellness) is the result of focused effort and expert advice (Hansen and Easthope forthcoming). For example Swinford and Webster describe wellness as 'being at your best' and achieving one's 'potential for wholeness and well-being' (Swinford and Webster 1989: 5). A rhetoric of empowerment and self-responsibility is a second point of commonality between holistic and wellness nursing and the new public health. This emphasis on self-empowerment means that holistic wellness nursing and the new public health can both appear attractive to nurses and clients who may both hope to escape the more traditional power relations of conventional medical care:

> It is significant that the new public health is frequently described as being a 'movement for change', and that it draws heavily on the language of many other new social movements, using terms such as 'self help', 'equity', 'access', 'collaboration', 'empowerment', 'participation', 'community control', and so on. The language has broad appeal, and its use has been an important means by which the new public health has achieved broad-based support while remaining closely wedded to official objectives.
>
> (Petersen and Lupton 1996: 11)

Closely linked to an expanded health concept and a focus on self-responsibility is a third area of similarity between the new public health and holistic/wellness nursing: a concern with monitoring and modifying individual lifestyles. The new public health, despite being described as an approach that moves beyond lifestyle, has a strong lifestyle focus and almost every aspect of living is seen as health related, including food, leisure, personal relationships, sun exposure, clothing, sex life, social support, housing, drug use and physical activity (Førde 1998; Nettleton 1995). Holistic and wellness nursing also place considerable emphasis on the importance of lifestyle (Leiby and Powelson 2003; Sieck et al. 2004).

For Bosch, holistic nursing is characterised by a 'reciprocal relationship between nurse and patient with emphasis on self responsibility, health promotion, and lifestyle' (Boschma 1994: 324). However, unlike the new public health where lifestyle factors are largely defined by epidemiological research into risk factors, holistic and wellness nursing expand available ideas about health-related lifestyle to include the emotions and spirituality. While the emphasis on spirituality in holistic wellness nursing has been influenced by Christian and pastoral nursing it also reflects the importance placed on spirituality in many CAM approaches (Cavendish et al. 2001; Pesut 2006).

Many CAM modalities place considerable focus on lifestyle (Schafer 1979; Storer et al. 1997). In CAM lifestyle is a very broad concept that may include factors such as attitude to living, energies and inter-personal relationships. There is frequently a strong focus on diet, digestion and exercise and on the importance of making informed and responsible choices in relation to these (Coward 1989: 11).

Despite a focus on healthy lifestyle practices, wellness nursing is, however, differentiated from normal health education or health promotion by a focus on individual wellness rather than population health risks, and by the use of 'wellness' rather than 'health' as a guiding concept. Even those aspects of wellness nursing that fall within the parameters of conventional health promotion display a concern with the emotional and psychosocial aspects of behaviours and behavioural change in a way that other public health texts do not (Faber and Rheinhardt 1982; Swinford and Webster 1989; Lunney 1993: 250).

Similarities between the new public health, wellness nursing and holistic nursing are not surprising. Nurses have been heavily involved in the construction and application of the new public health (Hansen and Easthope forthcoming). They are also key purveyors of health promotion and are frequently employed in public health roles (Petersen and Lupton 1996). Textbooks about health promotion and disease prevention written for and by nurses reflect a strong interest in the emotional and psychosocial aspects of behaviours and behavioural change (e.g. Faber and Rheinhardt 1982; Chin and Jacobs 1983) and nurses involved in health promotion and disease prevention can also be viewed as practitioners of the new public health (Hansen and Easthope forthcoming).

Furthermore, the new public health and holistic wellness nursing reproduce, and can themselves be seen as outputs of, the social and cultural conditions found in advanced Western societies in the second half of the twentieth century (Cant and Sharma 1999; Bauman 1992). Contemporary nursing understandings of lifestyle, health and disease reflect and reproduce a range of social processes that characterise the advanced industrialised societies of the late twentieth century (Giddens 1991). The most important of these inter-related processes and changes, in terms of their impact on holistic and wellness nursing, are 'the self as project' perspective associated with the ideology of conservative individualism (neoliberalism), the increasing commodification of health and health care, 'risk society' and population ageing. Each of these is discussed in turn below.

In contemporary societies 'one of the goals in life is to free oneself from social and cultural determination' (Gordon 1988: 34). Thus, the body is the site of choices and options that individuals must make in a reflexive manner (Giddens 1991: 8). Under these conditions health is viewed as an individual responsibility and a goal to be achieved as part of the ongoing project of enhancing the self. It is seen as a sign of 'competence, self control and self discipline' (Nettleton 1995: 50). This mode of thinking can be easily recognised in contemporary health policies, the new public health, CAM and in wellness and holistic nursing.

Related closely with the 'self as project' perspective is the commodification and commercialisation of bodies and health (Annandale 1998). As Turner explains, 'given the emphasis on selfhood in contemporary consumer culture the body is regarded as a changeable form of existence which can be shaped and which is malleable to individual needs and desires' (Turner 1996: 5). With the commodification of bodies, health becomes a commodity or possession that individuals can purchase. As a result, contemporary understandings of health and healthy lifestyles are inextricably interlinked with the rise of consumer culture (Featherstone 1991).

When health is viewed as a commodity to be purchased, Irvine argues, 'patients become consumers who "shop around" for health information' (Irvine 1999: 182). Sources of health-related information other than biomedicine come to be seen as valid and health-related advice becomes prevalent and profitable. The commodification of health has contributed to the growth of alternative therapies and the self-help and fitness industries (Easthope 2004). Along with a consumerist orientation come increased expectations about what medicine should actually offer patients (consumers). Thus provision of complementary therapies and preventive lifestyle advice is one aspect of the expanding medical package offered by doctors and nurses who find themselves in competition with other service providers such as pharmacists, naturopaths and physiotherapists.

A fourth process associated with rationality, individualism and commodification of late or high modernity is the 'risk society': where perceptions of risk are heightened and the identification and management of risks become a major concern (Beck 1992). Sociological arguments about a risk society emphasise that late/modern societies are characterised by a 'politics of anxiety' where the body is perceived as being under constant threat from external risks such as the destruction of the natural environment, chemical pollution and infections such as HIV/AIDS (Turner 1991). This social climate, which emphasises risks and the making of informed choices on the basis of knowledge, is reflected in an approach to health that defines healthy or unhealthy lifestyles in terms of lifestyle risks. Understanding the determinants of health or disease in terms of lifestyle risks 'advocates a rationalistic, individualistic, prospective life perspective where maximising control and minimising uncertainty is seen as a superior goal' (Førde 1998: 1155).

In addition to the influence of various processes and assumptions associated with late/high modernity, medical ideas and practices are also constructed though a nexus of demographic change and government policies on public health. In the mid- to late twentieth century improved living conditions resulted in a decline in infectious diseases and an increase in chronic conditions with behavioural and social determinants (Turner 1996). A growing elderly population in Western countries was predicted together with resultant issues related to an over-burdened health service and a shift in the disease burden. Short-term acute illness such as infections are replaced by the chronic diseases of the middle aged and elderly as major health problems. In response to these demographic changes, health policy-makers focused upon disease prevention as it became apparent that increasing investments in technological medicine resulted in diminishing returns (Turner 1996: 5). Policies and health education campaigns based on principles of disease prevention through individual lifestyle modification were widely implemented by governments in countries such as Australia, Canada and the United Kingdom (Palmer and Short 1994).

Relevance of the socio-cultural critique of the new public health for holistic and wellness nursing

The new public health has been subject to extensive socio-cultural critique (Nettleton and Bunton 1995). This critique is focused around the ways that the well-recognised normative components of public health are extended in the new public health.

> The new public health can be seen to involve much more than simply concern about 'health', as it is narrowly understood, or about achieving some 'essential' state of individual or collective well being and happiness. Above all, it is about the exercise of a particular form of power: one that presupposes and employs the regulated freedom of individuals to act in one way or the other.
>
> (Peterson and Lupton 1996: 26)

This critique has come primarily from sociology (although by the 1990s it was also apparent in some sociologically informed epidemiological, public health and health promotion textbooks and journal articles [e.g. Terris 1987; Bunton et al. 1995; Pearce 1996; Susser and Susser 1996; Wing 1994] and can be traced back to the 1970s when critics were concerned about the potential for victim blaming inherent in lifestyle-focused models of disease and the associated emphasis on self-responsibility [Crawford, 1978; Sontag, 1978]). The application of Foucauldian concepts of power/knowledge and panoptic surveillance and the increasing dominance of neo-liberalism as a discourse within the health arena increased the scope of this sociological critique (Petersen and Lupton 1996; Turner 1996). However, the new public health perspective is still hailed as a great advance in public health and disease prevention thinking by the majority of public health, health promotion and public health nursing texts and in government policies in countries such as Australia and the United Kingdom.

Three inter-related issues which are raised frequently within the socio-cultural critique are: that a focus on individual responsibility for health is moralistic and discriminatory; that the expanded biopsychosocial health concept found in the new public health increases the potential for medicalisation; and that this expanded concept reflects and reproduces the disciplinary powers of medicine through surveillance. Considering the many similarities (and differences) between the new public health and holistic wellness nursing outlined above, it is interesting to consider whether or not holistic wellness nursing is open to these same criticisms.

Is holistic wellness nursing potentially moralistic or discriminatory?

Within the sociocultural critique of the new public health it is assumed that models of disease which place individual lifestyle to the fore when explaining health and illness ('lifestyleism' or 'healthism') are fundamentally moralistic. Once health is linked with virtue, and becomes a seamless part of our ethical discourse, the regulation of lifestyle in the name of health acts as a mechanism for deterring vice and disciplining society. The underlying premise of a lifestyle approach is that 'good' behaviour will keep people healthy and that 'bad' behaviour will make them sick:

> Contained within what has come to be called the ideology of 'healthism' is a system of beliefs that defines health promoting activities, such as involvement in some form of physical fitness program as a moral obligation. Whether it is through exercise, diet, or stress management, the avoidance of disease through personal effort has become a dominant cultural motif.
>
> (White et al. 1995: 160)

Arguments about the inherent moralism of 'lifestyleism' have been focused on the ways that a healthy life is defined as an individual striving to reduce their risk of developing various diseases by participating in healthy activities. A healthy life is thus viewed as a virtuous life and illness suggests a failure to live a virtuous life – a phenomenon that has been termed victim-blaming. Disease or poor health is conceptualised in terms of individuals' non-compliance with the rules of a healthy lifestyle (Epstein 1995; Sontag 1989). An explanatory perspective that seeks to explain disease in terms of lifestyle is particularly problematic for those who develop a disease or condition that is apparently the direct result of something they did or did not do in their daily living (Horton and Aggleton 1989; Sontag 1978; 1989).

Another discriminatory aspect of an individualised lifestyle approach is the ways in which the approach focused on making lifestyle choices implies blame even though lifestyle risks are not equally distributed across the community. To argue that exposure to lifestyle risks is entirely the result of individual choice is discriminatory (Leichter 2003). Structural, behavioural and psychosocial determinants of health vary according to factors such as gender, geography, age, ethnicity and occupation. Members of low-income groups experience exclusion and a lack of control over their lives. A failure to recognise the links between material conditions and health-related risks is dishonest in terms of disease prevention (White 2002).

Learning to identify healthy activities and behaviours and assuming personal responsibility for health and wellness are key tenets of holistic well-ness nursing, the holistic nursing philosophy and associated CAM practices. For example, research projects conducted from a wellness perspective are frequently focused on recording behaviours such as alcohol consumption, cigarette smoking, exercise levels and types of activity, eating habits and uptake of medical screening tests such as pap smears in an attempt to develop wellness profiles. Research participants/clients are then advised about their wellness profile and offered advice and motivation to 'improve' their wellness (Ardell 1982; Nelson, et al. 2001; Paul and Weinert 1999). Thus it would seem that holistic wellness nursing can be described as poten-tially moralistic and judgemental. In the case of some holistic wellness texts the authors actually describe a wellness approach as being associated with moral development. For example, Swinford and Webster argue that a move towards wellness involves 'the evolving ability or maturity that the individual exercises in making decisions about what is right or wrong based on independent decision making and universal principles, including justice' (1989: 36).

The wellness nursing literature is also clearly focused on individuals and the frequently made statements about self-determinacy suggest a lack of recognition of the structural and socio-economic factors underpinning individual 'lifestyle choices' (Timmerman 1999). But, it is also clear in the literature that wellness is viewed as something that all people can strive for whatever their state of health; an individual who is in poor physical health (due to, for example, cardio-vascular disease) may also be viewed as working conscientiously towards wellness because he/she is involved in meditation, exercise and dietary modification. So, despite the facility for moralising, the use of wellness in place of health as a guiding concept may serve to reduce discrimination towards people who have already become sick.

Does holistic wellness nursing increase the potential for medicalisation?

The term medicalisation has come to refer to the complex process by which medicine is judged to be the appropriate social institution to deal with issues of disease and sickness. An increasing number of social issues come to be defined as illnesses or disorders and thus as medical problems. These social issues come to be defined as medical problems under medical governance, are described in medical language, understood in terms of a medical framework and are consequently managed via medical intervention (Conrad 1992). Examples of these processes or 'states of being' that have become included in the sphere of medical concern include life stages such as adolescence or old age, life events such as childbirth or pregnancy, and behaviours and practices such as alcoholism, fasting, binging and masturbation. Promiscuity, sadness, homosexuality and obesity have all at times been defined as disease states. Sociological writers have expressed concern about the problems associated with medicine substituting religion or the family as a major agent of social control (Conrad and Schneider 1980; Lupton 1997). However, other authors have argued that medicalisation should be viewed non-judgementally as a process which can be helpful in some contexts and destructive in others (Broom and Woodward 1996; Lowenberg and Davis 1994).

The new public health has been described as increasing the potential for medicalisation in two ways. First, the preventive focus on currently healthy people who might become unwell in the future increases the sphere of medical concern from states of illness to include health (Hughes 1994). Contemporary medical notions of lifestyle risk, where all people are required to consider their risk of disease even when they are currently healthy, places bodies in a state of transition where health is transformed into a state of 'virtual disease' (Hughes 1994). Second, if medicine utilises an approach towards disease that incorporates the social alongside the biological, then the self-limitation imposed by the biological reductionism of germ theory (the medical model) is removed and the sphere of possible medical influence is further increased. Lowenberg and Davis (1994) term this process, whereby the range of factors considered to be of importance to medicine is increased, an expansion of the pathogenic sphere.

Holistic wellness nursing provides an interesting case study in terms of medicalisation/demedicalisation. As part of a process of identifying clients' wellness profiles, facilitating their wellness goals and fostering self-care and self-awareness wellness practitioners have developed a set of nursing diagnoses known as wellness diagnoses. This is 'a type of nursing diagnosis that specifically relates to a situation where the patient is capable of promoting their state of health and wellness' (O'Connor and Parker 1995: 73). Such diagnoses are used by wellness practitioners in a process of health supervision where 'clients' are evaluated in order to identify practices, skills or attitudes that contribute to achieving wellness (Houldin et al. 1987; O'Connell 1996). Wellness-related diagnoses 'emphasize strengths that should be identified and enhanced to achieve the highest level of wellness possible for the client' (Houldin et al. 1987: v). Wellness diagnoses appear to provide a clear example of an expansion in the pathogenic sphere.

At the conceptual level wellness diagnoses use medical vocabulary to define a situation. Thus they appear to constitute part of a medicalising process whereby aspects of everyday life become classified medical and recorded as such (Houldin et al. 1987; Popkess-Vawter 1991; Stolte 1996; 1997). While wellness nurses make a point of defining a wellness diagnosis as a 'positive' diagnosis it is still defined in medical or technical language. Furthermore, the justification for making a wellness diagnosis is to create an opportunity for some type of nursing intervention even if simply to provide encouragement to 'keep up the good work' (Houldin et al. 1987). For example, Stolte (1997) describes using wellness diagnosis to record stages in the attainment of an appropriate maternal role by a young first time mother. She argues that the young mother in her study had not yet attained maternal attachment and the unspoken assumption is that she will require continued monitoring until she does achieve this state (Stolte 1997).

However, ambiguity remains about the relationship between holistic wellness diagnoses and medicalisation. Wellness diagnoses are clearly an example of nurses attempting to formalise their practices and have their professional skill included within the nursing lexicon despite the fact that nursing diagnoses may not be recognised as medical within the medical establishment and wellness diagnoses in particular are not well known outside of wellness nursing. In this case can they be classified as medical? Unfortunately because the medicalisation thesis has focused on medicine and doctors the place of nursing knowledge has been conflated with medical knowledge in general and thus this issue remains largely unexplored.

The use of CAM in holistic/wellness nursing further clouds this issue. The boundaries between medical knowledge and CAM (particularly certain CAM modalities such as homeopathy, massage, therapeutic touch and acupuncture) are not always clear (Shuval 2006; Hollenberg 2006; May and Sirur 1998; Easthope 1999). Wellness nurses are practising as nurses focusing on people who while called clients are in fact patients and using CAM and wellness diagnoses as part of their work and as such do count as part of medicine and thus fall under the medicalisation critique.

Does holistic wellness nursing contribute to surveillance and the disciplinary power of medicine?

Medical sociologists who adopt a Foucauldian perspective have focused on the body as a target of disciplinary practices and extended the medicalisation critique to argue that the programmes and technologies of health promotion contribute to 'an increasingly all encompassing network of surveillance and observation' (Nettleton and Bunton 1995: 47). Such authors draw on Foucault's writings about disciplinary power and his concept of panoptic surveillance to examine 'the ways in which forms of governance involve the investigation and regulation of the body of the individual and bodies of populations' (Nettleton and Bunton 1995: 47).

There are two aspects to the surveillance critique of the new public health. The first focuses on how the new public health reflects a displacement of the traditional medical site of surveillance, the clinic, by the discursive space of epidemiology and the related technologies of health promotion and health education (Turner 1996; Williams 1998: 448). From this perspective the disciplinary powers of medicine have been increased by the adoption of what Armstrong calls 'social medicine' (Armstrong 1983: 38). Disease prevention measures that focus on altering lifestyles are viewed as evidence of the 'growing penetration of the clinical gaze into the everyday lives of citizens, including their emotional states, the nature of their interpersonal relationships, the management of stress and other lifestyle choices' (Lupton 1997: 107).

The second aspect of the surveillance critique addresses the inter-relationship between institutional dictates on bodily management and every-day life for individuals (Lupton 1997: 103). The new public health places emphasis on self-control, self-discipline and self-monitoring of lifestyle risks and as such surveillance is carried out by individuals as they assess their own bodies, states of health or sickness and ways of living in terms of medical/public health advice about lifestyle (Glassner 1989).

The surveillance argument can be applied to holistic wellness nursing and holistic nursing in general. A holistic nursing approach encourages nurses to move beyond their sick patients' bodies to consider the bodies of healthy patients/clients and their emotions, feelings and thoughts. This is a practice that in other contexts 'could be regarded as an invasion of an individual's privacy' but in the context of holistic medical care 'it is generally accepted as appropriate and even important' (Lupton 2002: 186).

In addition, holistic wellness nursing is an approach often applied in the context of public health nursing and health promotion. These nursing areas are dominated by individual level interventions like lifestyle coun-selling and home visits to 'at risk' clients such as teenage single mothers or the chronically ill (Grumbach et al. 2004). The public health and health promotion aspects of wellness nursing involve disciplinary powers of 'observation, examination, measurement and the comparison of individuals against an established norm, bringing them into a field of visibility' (Lupton 1997: 99).

Furthermore, the holistic health focus on self-responsibility is a demonstration of the second aspect of the surveillance critique whereby individuals exert disciplinary powers over themselves. Wellness is seen as a process and as something to strive for. Thus patient/clients are being trained to monitor and assess their own behaviours and actions in terms of their relationship to wellness. Holistic wellness nurses describe their role as one where they actively encourage their patients/clients to live a 'wellness lifestyle' through critically examining and monitoring their own health-related risk factors (Chambers-Clark 1986; Kickbusch and Payne 2003). Fromm and Trustem (1989) describe a long list of 'self responsible health behaviours' that make up part of a wellness lifestyle. These include periodic physician check-ups, breast self-examination, testicular self-examination and colorectal screening every three to five years (Fromm and Trustem 1989).

Discussion

Holistic wellness nursing and the new public health share many points of similarity. Those discussed in this chapter include a biopsychosocial understanding of health, a focus on lifestyles and an emphasis on individual responsibility for health. Similarities between holistic health and conventional medicine and public health perspectives have been observed by a number of writers (Wolpe 1990; May and Sirur 1998; Montgomery 1993).

Nursing was an influential discipline in the social construction of the new public health and at times it is difficult to confidently distinguish between the new public health and holistic wellness nursing. Indeed, since many wellness nurses practise in the fields of health promotion, disease prevention, and public health, they may in fact be working within the new public health. Despite the clear biomedical underpinnings of the new public health and the strong CAM influences in holistic wellness nursing both are arguably part of the same larger processes of neoliberalism and reflexive modernity (Featherstone 1991).

Due to the overlap between holistic wellness nursing and some aspects of the new public health, the socio-cultural critique of the new public health can be applied to holistic wellness nursing. Three aspects of the critique and its application to holistic wellness nursing have been explored in this chapter. First, that models of health and disease that emphasise self-responsibility for health are moralistic and potentially discriminatory. Second, that biopsychosocial understandings of health extend medicalisation, and third, that the technologies of public health and health promotion extend the disciplinary powers of medicine and increase opportunities for bodily surveillance and control.

As demonstrated throughout the chapter, each of these arguments is relevant to holistic wellness nursing. Some aspects of holistic wellness nursing reveal a frightening advance of surveillance, medicalisation and the potential for victim-blaming. With the concept of wellness, holistic wellness nursing arguably increases the scope of health beyond the physical and behavioural to include the emotional and spiritual. Even so, the claim that the socio-cultural critique of the new public health holds equally true for holistic wellness nursing should be viewed with some reservations.

At least three issues impact on how well the socio-cultural critique can be applied to holistic wellness nursing. First, there is considerable variation in the use of different CAM modalities among holistic nurses as there is among the various CAM approaches that they use (Hirschkorn and Bourgeault 2005: 157). Further empirical research of nurses who identify themselves as holistic and as wellness practitioners is required to bear this out (Hirschkorn and Bourgeault 2005; Tovey and Adams 2003; Shuval 2006). Next, there is also a difference in scope between the new public health and wellness nursing: wellness nursing is focused on individuals not populations and although the new public health is applied at the level of individuals it is generally a policy response directed at populations. Third, there are continuities between the theory and practice of wellness nursing that are not present between the theory and application of the new public health. To take up this last point of difference, the theory of the new public health, argue authors such as Hughes (1994) and Petersen and Lupton (1996), contains a number of attractive features but in application often amounts to little more than lecturing people about how they live, which when encoded in programmes, affords governments the opportunity to shift responsibility for health into the hands of individual citizens while neglecting the structural and material factors underpinning patterns of health and illness and lifestyle 'choices'. The theory of holistic wellness nursing, on the other hand, can often appear moralistic but is likely to be far more flexible in application. Holistic wellness nurses primarily work with individuals and do so at an inter-personal level. Research investigating holistic practitioners has found that while they offer general theoretical explanations for disease that imply individuals are responsible for their own health, they are often reluctant to describe their own patients as being personally responsible for ill-health (Lowenberg and Davis 1994).

McClean contends that by personalising and individualising health and illness CAM approaches engage 'the individuality of the person' (2005: 635). While this could be understood in terms of victim-blaming, CAM can also be understood in terms of empowering healers and patients by providing them 'with greater agency and control in the construction of healing reality' (McClean 2005: 644). Perhaps holistic wellness nursing can be understood in a parallel way? However, this goes to the question of whether nursing is the appropriate profession to deal with emotional and spiritual well-being through CAM. It may be that wellness nursing offers a valuable contribution to individual flourishing but that the institutional status of nursing (as a paramedical profession) makes the practice of wellness nursing and CAM morally perilous. Holistic wellness nursing does place CAM in an invidious position with regard to medicine. The adoption of non-medical discourses into nursing theory especially given the clinical setting of much nursing practice provides greater possibilities for oppression. There is a difference between opening a space in which others can themselves pursue health and wellness and disciplining others with potentially oppressive representations of a healthy or well self, which is blurred in the institutional or clinical setting. Perhaps a greater awareness among nurses of the socio-cultural critique of the new public health and the relevance of this critique for holistic wellness nursing will serve to stimulate debate among holistic wellness nurses about these complicated and important issues.

References

Adams, J. (2004) Demarcating the medical/non-medical border: occupational boundary-work within GPs' accounts of their integrative practice. In Tovey, P., Easthope, G. and Adams, J. (eds) *The Mainstreaming of Complementary and Alternative Medicine: Studies in Social Context*, London and New York: Routledge, pp. 140–57.

Adams, J. (2006) An exploratory study of complementary and alternative medicine in hospital midwifery: models of care and professional struggle. *Complementary Therapies in Clinical Practice* 12(1): 40–7.

Adams, J. and Tovey, P. (2001) Nurses' use of professional distancing in the appropriation of CAM. *Complementary Therapies in Medicine* 9(3): 136–40.

Allen, C. (1991) Holistic concepts and the professionalization of public health nursing. *Public Health Nursing* 8(2): 74–80.

Annandale, E. (1998) *The Sociology of Health and Medicine*. Cambridge: Polity Press.

Anspaugh, D. J., Hamrick, M. H. and Rosato, F. D. (1994) *Wellness: Concepts and Applications*. St Louis, MD: C. V. Mosby Company.

Ardell, D. (1982) *Fourteen Days to a Wellness Lifestyle*. Mill Valley, CA: Whatever Publishing Co.

Armstrong, D. (1983). *The Political Anatomy of the Body: Medical Knowledge in the Twentieth Century*. Cambridge: Cambridge University Press.

Ashton, J. and Seymour, H. (1988) *The New Public Health: The Liverpool Experience*. Milton Keynes: Open University Press.

Auger, S. (1990) Nursing Practice and Holism. *International Review of Community Development* 24(64): 57–9.

Bacon, L., Keim, N. L., Van Loan, M. D., Derricote, M., Gale, B., Kazaks, A. and Stern, J. S. (2002) Evaluating a 'non-diet' wellness intervention for improvement of metabolic fitness, psychological well-being and eating and activity behaviours. *International Journal of Obesity* 26(6): 854–65.

Baer, H. (2004) *Toward an Integrative Medicine: Merging Alternative Therapies with Biomedicine.* Walnut Creek, CA: Altamira Press.

Bauman, Z. (1992) *Intimations of Postmodernity.* London: Routledge.

Beck, U. (1992) *Risk Society: Towards a New Modernity.* London: Sage.

Boschma, G. (1994) The meaning of holism in nursing: historical shifts in holistic nursing ideas. *Public Health Nursing* 11(5): 324–30.

Broom, D. and Woodward, R. V. (1996) Medicalisation reconsidered: towards a collaborative approach to care. *Sociology of Health and Illness* 18(3): 357–78.

Bunton, R., Nettleton, S. and Burrows, R. (eds) (1995) *The Sociology of Health Promotion: Critical Analysis of Consumption, Lifestyle and Risk.* London: Routledge.

Cant, S. and Sharma, U. (1999) *A New Medical Pluralism? Alternative Medicine, Doctors and the State.* London: UCL Press.

Cant, S. and Sharma, U. (2000) Alternative health practices and systems. In Albrecht, G. L., Fitzpatrick, R. and Scrimshaw, S. (eds) *Handbook of Social Studies in Health and Medicine.* Thousand Oaks, CA: Sage, pp. 426–39.

Cavendish, R., Luise, B. and Horne, K. (2001) Recognising opportunities for enhancing spirituality relevant to young adults. *Nursing Diagnosis* 12: 77–91.

Chambers-Clark, C. C. (1986). *Wellness Nursing: Concepts, Theory, Research and Practice.* New York: Springer Publishing Company.

Chin, P. and Jacobs, M. (1983) *Theory and Nursing: A Systematic Approach.* St Louis, MD: C. V. Mosby Company.

Cohen, M. Z. and Bumbaugh, M. (2004) Group dream work: a holistic resource for oncology nurses. *Oncology Nursing Forum* 31(4): 817–24.

Conrad, P. (1992) Medicalisation and social control. *Annual Review of Sociology* 18: 209–32.

Conrad, P. and Schneider, J. W. (1980) *Deviance and Medicalisation: From Badness to Sickness.* St Louis, MD: C. V. Mosby Company.

Coward, R. (1989) *The Whole Truth: The Myth of Alternative Medicine.* London: Faber and Faber.

Crawford, R. (1978) You are dangerous to your health: the ideology and politics of victim blaming. *Social Policy* 8(4): 10–20.

Drewnowski, A., Monsen, E., Birkett, D., Gunther, S., Vendeland, S., Su, J. and Marshall, G. (2003) Health screening and health promotion programs for the elderly. *Disease Management & Health Outcomes* 11(5): 299–309.

Easthope, G. (1999) The response of orthodox medicine to the challenge of alternative medicine in Australia. *Australian and New Zealand Journal of Sociology* 29(3): 289–301.

Easthope, G. (2004) Consuming health: the market for complementary and alternative medicine. *Australian Journal of Primary Health Care* 10(2): 68–75.

Epstein, J. (1995) *Altered Conditions: Disease, Medicine and Storytelling.* New York: Routledge.

Faber, M. and Rheinhardt, A. (1982) *Promoting Health Through Risk Reduction.* New York: Macmillan.

Featherstone, M. (1991) *Consumer Culture and Postmodernism.* London: Sage.

Fenton, M. V. and Morris, D. L. (2003) The integration of holistic nursing practices and complementary and alternative modalities into curricula of schools of nursing. *Alternative Therapies in Health and Medicine* 9(4): 62–7.

Ford, P. and McCormack, B. (2000) Keeping the person in the centre of nursing. *Nursing Standard* 14(46): 40–4.

Førde, O. (1998) Is imposing risk awareness cultural imperialism? *Social Science & Medicine* 47(9): 1155–9.

Frisch, N. C. (2003) Standards of holistic nursing practice as guidelines for quality undergraduate nursing curricula. *Journal of Professional Nursing* 19(6): 382–6.

Fromm, C. G. and Trustem, A. (1989) Self-responsibility. In Swinford, P. A. and Webster, J. A. (eds) *Promoting Wellness: A Nurse's Handbook*. Rockville, MD: Aspen Publishers.

Fullagar, S. (2002) Governing the healthy body: discourses of leisure and lifestyle within Australian health policy. *Health* 6(1): 69–84.

Giasson, M. and Bouchard, L. (1998) Effect of therapeutic touch on the well-being of persons with terminal cancer. *Journal of Holistic Nursing* 16(3): 383–98.

Giddens, A. (1991) *Modernity and Self Identity*. Oxford: Polity Press.

Glassner, B. (1989) Fitness and the postmodern self. *Journal of Health and Social Behaviour* 30(2): 180–91.

Gordon, D. (1988) Tenacious assumptions in Western medicine. In Lock, M. and Gordon, D. (eds) *Biomedicine Examined*. Dortrecht: Kluwer Academic Publishers.

Greenberg, J. S., Dintiman, G. B. and Oakes, B .M. (1997) *Wellness: Creating a Life of Health and Fitness*. Boston, MA: Allyn and Bacon.

Grumbach, K., Miller, J., Mertz, E. and Finocchio, L. (2004) How much public health in public health nursing practice? *Public Health Nursing* 21(3): 266–76.

Hansen, E. C. and Easthope, G. (forthcoming) *Lifestyle in Medicine*. London: Routledge.

Helms, J. E. (2006) Complementary and alternative therapies: a new frontier for nursing education. *Journal of Nursing Education* 45(3): 117–23.

Hirschkorn, K. and Bourgeault, I. (2005) Conceptualizing mainstream health care providers' behaviours in relation to complementary and alternative medicine. *Social Science & Medicine* 61(1): 157–70.

Hoffmann, F. L. (1991) Feminism and nursing. *The National Woman Studies Association Journal* 3(1): 53–69.

Hollenberg, D. (2006) Uncharted ground: patterns of professional interaction among complementary/alternative and biomedical practitioners in integrative health care settings. *Social Science & Medicine* 62(3): 731–44.

Hoover, J. (2002) The personal and professional impact of undertaking an educational module on human caring. *Journal of Advanced Nursing* 37(1): 79–86.

Horton, M. and Aggleton, P. (1989) Perverts, inverts and experts: the cultural production of the AIDS research paradigm. In Aggleton, P., Hart, G. and Davies, P. (eds) *AIDS: Social Representations, Social Practices*. London: The Falmer Press, pp. 74–100.

Houldin, A. D., Saltstein, S. W. and Ganley, K. M. (1987) *Nursing Diagnoses for Wellness: Supporting Strengths*. Philadelphia, PA: J. B. Lippincott Company.

Hughes, M. (1994) The risks of lifestyle and the diseases of civilisation. *Annual Review of Health Social Sciences* 4: 57–78.

Irvine, R. (1999) Losing patients: health care, consumers, power and sociocultural change. In Grbich, C. (ed.) *Health in Australia: Sociological Concepts and Issues.* Sydney: Prentice Hall, pp. 191–214.

Johnson, M. B. (1990) The holistic paradigm in nursing: the diffusion of an innovation. *Research in Nursing and Health* 13: 129–39.

Kickbusch, I. and Payne, L. (2003) Twenty-first century health promotion: the public health revolution meets the wellness revolution. *Health Promotion International* 18(4): 275–8.

King, M. Q. and Gates, M. F. (2006) Perceived barriers to holistic nursing in undergraduate nursing programs. *The Journal of Science and Healing* 2(4): 334–8.

Leiby, K. and Powelson, S. (2003) Potential for enhanced exercise: a study of wellness in college students. *International Journal of Nursing Termininologies and Classifications* 14(4) Supplement October–December: 48.

Leichter, H. M. (2003) 'Evil habits' and 'personal choices': assigning responsibility for health in the 20th century. *Milbank Quarterly* 81(4): 603–26.

Lowdon, B., Davis, D., Ferguson, P., Dickie, B., and Marron, K. (1993) *Wellness.* Geelong: Deakin University.

Lowenberg, J. (1989) *Caring and Responsibility: The Crossroads between Holistic Practice and Traditional Medicine.* Philadelphia, PA: University of Philadelphia Press.

Lowenberg, J. S. and Davis, F. (1994) Beyond medicalisation-demedicalisation: the case of holistic health. *Sociology of Health and Illness* 16(5): 579–99.

Lunney, J. (1993) Development of a program of health promotion research. In Wilson-Barnett, J. and Macleod-Clark, J. (eds) *Research in Health Promotion.* London: Macmillan, pp. 63–78.

Lupton, D. (1997) Foucault and the medicalisation critique. In Petersen, A. and Bunton, R. (eds) *Foucault, Health and Medicine* London: Routledge, pp. 94–110.

Lupton, D. (2002) The body, medicine and society. In Germov, J. (ed.) *Second Opinion: An Introduction to Health Sociology.* Melbourne: Oxford University Press, pp. 121–36.

McClean, S. (2005) 'The illness is part of the person': discourses of blame, individual responsibility and individuation at a centre for spiritual healing in the North of England. *Sociology of Health and Illness* 27(5): 628–48.

McCoppin, B. and Gardner, H. (1994) *Tradition and Reality: Nursing and Politics in Australia.* Melbourne: Churchill Livingstone.

May, C. and Sirur, D. (1998). Art, science and placebo: incorporating homepathy in general practice. *Sociology of Health and Illness* 20(2): 186–90.

Montgomery, S. (1993) Illness and image in holistic discourse: how alternative is alternative? *Cultural Critique* 25: 65–89.

Nelson, G., Laurendeau, M. C. and Chamberland, C. (2001) A review of programs to promote family wellness and prevent the maltreatment of children. *Canadian Journal of Behavioural Science-Revue* 33(1): 1–13.

Nettleton, S. (1995) *The Sociology of Health and Illness.* Cambridge: Polity Press.

Nettleton, S. and Bunton, R. (1995) Sociological critiques of health promotion. In Bunton, R. and Nettleton, S. (eds) *The Sociology of Health Promotion: Critical Analysis of Consumption, Lifestyle and Risk.* London: Routledge, pp. 41–58.

O'Connell, B. (1996) Nursing process: a systematic approach to patient care. In Greenwood, J. (ed.) *Nursing Theory in Australia: Development and Application.* Sydney: Harper Educational.

O'Connor, M. L. and Parker, E. (1995) *Health Promotion: Principles and Practice in the Australian Context.* St Leonards NSW: Allen and Unwin.

Palmer, G. R. and Short, S. D. (1994) *Health Care and Public Policy: An Australian Analysis.* Melbourne: Macmillan Education Australia.

Paul, L. and Weinert, C. (1999) Wellness profile of midlife women with a chronic illness. *Public Health Nursing* 16(5): 341–50.

Pearce, N. (1996) Traditional epidemiology, modern epidemiology and public health. *American Journal of Public Health* 86(5): 678–83.

Pender, N. J. (1982) *Health Promotion in Nursing Practice.* Norwalk CT: Appleton-Century Crofts.

Pesut, B. (2006) Fundamental of foundational obligations? Problematising the ethical call to spiritual care in nursing. *Advances in Nursing Science* 29(2): 125–32.

Petersen, A. and Lupton, D. (1996) *The New Public Health: Health and Self in the Age of Risk.* St Leonards NSW: Allen and Unwin.

Petosa, R. (1984) Wellness: an emerging opportunity for health education. *Health Education* 15(6): 37–9.

Plawecki, H. M. (1996) Editorial: the advancement of holistic nursing practice. *Journal of Holistic Nursing* 14(2): 83–4.

Popkess-Vawter, S. (1991) Wellness nursing diagnoses: to be or not to be? *Nursing Diagnosis* 2(1): 19–25.

Schafer, R. (1979) The self-concept factor in diet selection and quality. *Journal of Nutrition Education* 11: 37–9.

Shuval, J. (2006) Nurses in alternative health care: integrating medical paradigms. *Social Science & Medicine* 63(7): 1784–95.

Siahpush, M. (1998) Postmodern values, dissatisfaction with conventional medicine and popularity of alternative therapies. *Journal of Sociology* 34(1): 56–70.

Sieck, C. J., Heirich, M. and Major, C. (2004) Alcohol counseling as part of general wellness counseling. *Public Health Nursing* 21(2): 137–43.

Slater, V. E., Maloney, J. P., Krau, S. D. and Eckert, C. A. (1999) Journey to holism. *Journal of Holistic Nursing* 17(4): 365–83.

Sontag, S. (1978) *Illness as Metaphor.* New York: Farrar, Strauss and Giroux.

Sontag, S. (1989) *Illness as Metaphor/AIDS and its Metaphors.* New York: Anchor Publishing.

Stolte, K. M. (1996) *Wellness Nursing Diagnosis For Health Promotion.* Philadelphia, PA: Lippincott-Raven Publishers.

Stolte, K. M. (1997) Wellness nursing diagnosis: accentuating the positive. *American Journal of Nursing* 97(7): 16B–16N.

Storer, J. H., Cychosz, C. M. and Anderson, D. F. (1997) Wellness behaviours, social identities and health promotion. *The American Journal of Health Behaviour* 21(4): 260–8.

Susser, M. and Susser, E. (1996) Choosing a future for epidemiology: eras and paradigms. *American Journal of Public Health* 86: 668–73.

Swinford, P. A. and Webster, J. A. (1989) *Promoting Wellness: A Nurse's Handbook*. Rockville, MD: Aspen Publishers.

Terris, M. (1987) Epidemiology and the public health movement. *Journal of Public Health Policy* 8(3): 315.

Timmerman, G. M. (1999) Using self-care strategies to make lifestyle changes. *Journal of Holistic Nursing* 17(2): 169–83.

Tovey, P. and Adams, J. (2003) Nostalgic and nostophobic referencing and the authentication of nurses' use of complementary therapies. *Social Science & Medicine* 56(7): 1469–80.

Turner, B. S. (1991) Recent developments in the theory of the body. In Featherstone, M., Hepworth, M. and Turner, B. S. (eds) *The Body: Social Process and Cultural Theory*. London: Sage, pp. 1–35.

Turner, B. S. (1996) *The Body and Society*. London: Sage.

White, K. (2002) *An Introduction to the Sociology of Health and Illness*. London: Sage.

White, P., Young, K. and Gillett, J. (1995) Bodywork as a moral imperative: some critical notes on health and fitness. *Society and Leisure* 18(1): 159–82.

WHO (World Health Organization) (1986) *Ottowa Charter*. Copenhagen: Regional Office For Europe.

Williams, S. J. (1998) Health as moral performance: ritual transgression and taboo. *Health* 2(4): 435–57.

Wing, S. (1994) Limits of epidemiology. *Medicine and Global Survival* 1: 74–86.

Wolpe, P. R. (1990) The holistic heresy: strategies of ideological challenge in the medical profession. *Social Science & Medicine* 31(8): 913–23.

Wong, R., Sagar, C. M. and Sagar, S. M. (2001) Integration of Chinese Medicine into supportive cancer care: a modern role for an ancient tradition. *Cancer Treatment Review* 27(4): 235–46.

Woods, C. Q. (1987) From individual dedication to social activism: historical development of nursing professionalism. In Maggs, C. (ed.) *Nursing History: The State of the Art*. London: Croom Helm, pp. 153–75.

Zengerle-Levy, K. (2004) Practices that facilitate critically burned children's holistic healing. *Qualitative Health Research* 14(9): 1255–75.

Index